HUNGRY
FOR
CHANGE

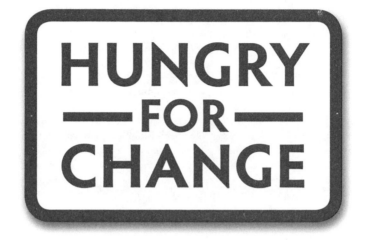

HUNGRY —FOR— CHANGE

Ditch the Diets, Conquer the Cravings, and Eat Your Way to Lifelong Health

James Colquhoun and Laurentine ten Bosch

HarperOne
An Imprint of HarperCollins*Publishers*

HarperOne

All images, with the exception of pages 1 and 260, are reprinted
from the film *HUNGRY FOR CHANGE* by permission.
Page 1: Photograph by Lizz Pennings.
Page 260: "EWG's 2012 Shoppers Guide to Pesticides in Produce"
reprinted by permission of the Environmental Working Group.

HarperCollins books may be purchased for educational,
business, or sales promotional use. For information, please e-mail the
Special Markets Department at SPsales@harpercollins.com.

HarperCollins website: http://www.harpercollins.com

HarperCollins®, 🏭®, and HarperOne™ are trademarks
of HarperCollins Publishers.

FIRST EDITION

Designed by Terry McGrath

Library of Congress Cataloging-in-Publication Data

Colquhoun, James.
Hungry for change : ditch the diets, conquer the cravings, and eat your way to
lifelong health / by James Colquhoun, Laurentine ten Bosch. — 1st ed.
p. cm.
ISBN 978–0–06–222084–4
1. Weight loss. 2. Health. 3. Nutrition. 4. Lifestyles—Health aspects.
I. Bosch, Laurentine ten. II. Title.
RM222.2.C572   2012
613.2'5—dc23   2012023456

12 13 14 15 16 RRD(H) 10 9 8 7 6 5 4 3 2 1

This book is dedicated to that part within all of us that strives for perfect health, our innate birthright.

Contents

PART II: YOUR HEALTH IS IN YOUR HANDS

Foreword

The Last Diet You Will Ever Need

Why do we believe that we can feed our bodies manufac-tured, nutrient-depleted, food-like substances, empty of all life, and yet remain healthy? How did we come to believe that industrial chemicals and processing could replace what nature produces? A hundred years ago, all food was organic, local, seasonal, and fresh or naturally preserved by ancient methods. All food was food. Now, less than 3 percent of agricultural land in the United States is used to grow fruits and vegetables, which should make up 80 percent of our diets. Today, not even enough fruits and vegetables are grown in this country to allow all Americans to eat the five to nine servings a day set forth by the U.S. government's dietary guidelines.

What most of us are left with is industrial food. And who knows what lurks in the average boxed, packaged, or canned factory-made science project. When a French fry has more than 20 ingredients and almost all of them are not potatoes, when a fast food hamburger con-tains very little meat, and when the average teenager consumes 34 teaspoons of sugar each day, we are living in a food nightmare, a sci-fi horror show.

The very fact that we are having a national conversation about what we should eat, that we are struggling with how to define the "best" diet, is symptomatic of how far we have strayed from the natural conditions that gave rise to our species and from the simple act of eating real, whole, fresh food. When eating real food is a revolutionary act, we are in trouble.

The food industry—which is the second-largest employer in the United States, after the federal government, and which heavily influences both the media and the government agencies that regulate it (the Department of Agriculture, the Food and Drug Administration, and Congress)—intentionally confuses and confounds us. Low-fat is good, so anything with "low-fat" on the label must be healthy. But a soda is 100 percent fat-free, and that doesn't make it healthy. Now we are being told to eat more whole grains, so a few flecks of whole grains have been sprinkled on sugary cereals. That doesn't make them healthy either. The best advice is to avoid foods with health claims on their labels. Better yet, avoid foods with labels in the first place.

Our taste buds, our brain chemistry, our biochemistry, our hormones, and our kitchens have been hijacked by the food industry. The food-like substances proffered by the industrial food system trick our taste buds into momentary pleasure but not our biology, which reacts, rejects, and reviles the junk plied on our genes and our hormonal and biochemical pathways. We need to "unjunk" our biology.

Industrial processing has given rise to an array of addictive, fattening, metabolism-jamming chemicals and compounds, including MSG (monosodium glutamate), aspartame, high-fructose corn syrup, and trans fats, to name the biggest offenders. Researchers use MSG to study obesity. It is an "excitotoxin" that stimulates the brain into wanting to eat uncontrollably. When fed to laboratory mice, the mice pig out and get fat. MSG is in 80 percent of all processed foods, mostly disguised as a "natural flavoring." Trans fats, another example, are derived from vegetable oils and then chemically altered to resist degradation by bacteria, which is why store-bought cookies can last on your pantry shelf for years. But the ancient energy system of our body's cells is descended from bacteria, and those mitochondria cannot process trans fats. Our metabolism becomes blocked, and weight gain and type 2 diabetes ensue.

Our tongues can be fooled by and our brains can become addicted to the slick combinations of fat, sugar, and salt pumped into factory-made foods, but our biochemistry cannot, and the result is the disaster of obesity and chronic disease that we have in the United States today.

It is no wonder that 68 percent of Americans are overweight and that, since 1960, the obesity rate has risen from 13 percent to 36 percent and soon will reach 42 percent. Over the last decade, the rate of prediabetes or diabetes in teenagers has risen from 9 percent to 23 percent. Really? Almost one in four of our kids now has either prediabetes or type 2 diabetes. And 37 percent of the kids who are not considered overweight have one or more cardiovascular risk factors, such as high blood pressure, high cholesterol, or high blood sugar, because even though factory food hasn't yet made them fat, it is making them sick!

It is time to take our kitchens and our homes back. Transforming the food industry seems a monumental undertaking. But it is not. It is a small problem. It is in the small places of our lives: in our shopping carts, our fridges, our cupboards, our kitchens, and our dining rooms. This is where all of our power is. The hundreds of little choices we make every day can topple the monolithic food industry. The past century is littered with the remains of fallen despots and despotic regimes. From the fall of the Berlin Wall to the rise of the Arab Spring, there is no force more powerful than a small group of individuals with a desire to end injustice and abuse.

HUNGRY FOR CHANGE breaks through any confusion about what is in the food we eat today and plants the seeds of revolution with very simple ideas: Our bodies were designed to run on real food. Our natural state is health. We need to simplify our ways of eating. If we unjunk our diets and detoxify our bodies and minds, we heal. Simply choose real food: vegetables, fruits, nuts, seeds, healthy oils (olive, fish, avocado, and coconut), and small amounts of whole grains, beans, and lean animal proteins, including wild-caught fish, organic grass-fed meats, and organic free-range eggs.

In this book, there is no diet regimen, no calorie counting, and no measuring of fats, carbs, or protein grams. None of that matters if you choose real, whole, fresh, live foods. If you choose quality, the rest takes care of itself. When you eat empty industrial foods, with their addictive chemicals and sugars, your body craves more because it needs nutrients not found in dead foods. Yet after eating nutrient-dense fresh foods for a few days, you break the biological addiction to industrial foods. After a few more days, your cells begin to rejuvenate and your body heals from the inside out. And the side effects are all good ones: effortless weight loss; a reversal of high blood pressure, diabetes, and high cholesterol; a clearing of any foggy headedness; a lifting of depression and fatigue; and healthier skin, hair, and nails.

More important than what you take out of your diet is what you put into it. Add in the good stuff and there won't be room for the bad. Mother Nature is the best pharmacist, and real food is the most powerful drug on the planet. Real food works faster, better, and cheaper than any pharmaceutical. And when spiced up with a few superfoods, such as chia seeds, hemp seeds, parsley, cilantro, coconut, and green juices, a diet of whole real food can benefit thousands of genes, regulate dozens of hormones, and enhance the function of tens of thousands of protein networks. Dinner becomes your date with the doctor. What you put at the end of your fork is more powerful than anything you will ever find at the bottom of a prescription bottle.

HUNGRY FOR CHANGE offers us a simple road map to health. Real food, adequate sleep and physical movement, self-love rather than self-loathing, and holding on to a healthy image of yourself—solutions to both our health crisis and our obesity epidemic are not complicated. Health and happiness are often just a few days away. Plus, by making small changes in our lives, each of us has the capacity to effect big changes in our food landscape, our agriculture system, and even government policies. I hope *HUNGRY FOR CHANGE* is the start of a true food revolution.

Mark Hyman, M.D.
West Stockbridge, Massachusetts
May 29, 2012

Introduction: Our Story

Our story begins with our family. In 2003, my father, Roy, was diagnosed with chronic fatigue syndrome, or CFS. CFS is called a syndrome because the cause and the cure are unknown. At the time, we didn't realize how much this was going to impact all of our lives. We thought we could outsource treatment to the medical profession and move on. How wrong we were.

For the next five years, Roy's days were spent in bed, and his nights were often filled with sweaty panic attacks, the anticipated side effects

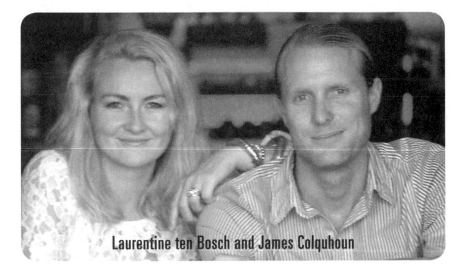

Laurentine ten Bosch and James Colquhoun

of his medications. The vicious cycle continued as Roy was on two to three medications for his condition and another two to three medications to curb the side effects. He had gained more than 55 pounds and was increasingly lethargic.

Seeing Roy's health deteriorate was a painful experience for us as a family. He was no longer the energetic, driven, active man we had known throughout our lives. Before he was diagnosed with CFS, Roy was a professional accountant, tax adviser, and business owner. He had significant financial responsibilities advising companies and high-net-worth individuals. His daily routine consisted of intense and long work hours, eating on the run, lots of sugar and coffee, and in true Australian fashion, plenty of beers with his mates after a hard day at the office.

To counteract his high-stress, fast-paced life, Roy, like many of us, looked to fat-free products and diet sodas—anything that seemed even remotely healthy. He understood that his job was taxing his health, and he was looking for a way to counterbalance the effects. As long as it was marketed as a "health" product or was recommended by a doctor, it was on our table.

When the physical and mental demands of Roy's job finally caught up with him, he sought the advice of medical professionals, just as we're all taught to do. Roy was gaining weight and having trouble both getting up in the morning and getting to sleep at night. He felt tired all day long. He met with many doctors, including our family's longtime general practitioner. They immediately prescribed a course of medications. Not one suggested he change his diet or eating habits or recommended different ways to handle stress. Their advice: take the pills, and we'll see how it goes.

Not surprisingly, Roy's health began to deteriorate further. He continued to consult with his doctors, who prescribed more and more medications. They were determined to try different "cocktails" to figure out which magic combination would work. He remained hopeful that the doctors would find a chemical solution. He had no reason to believe otherwise.

Eventually, however, Roy had to sell his business. It was a sad day—for him and for all of us. This company had been a driving purpose and mission in his life, and as he let it go, he felt that he was giving up a part of himself, a part of his identity. At the same time, his condition continued to worsen, and the emotional impact of the loss of his business led to chronic depression and severe anxiety. The more medications he took, the worse he became.

Laurentine and I knew we had to intervene. We had always taken an interest in nutrition and health and had shared our then limited knowledge with Roy. But every attempt to help was met with keen resistance. "These doctors have spent their entire lives training to help me. What makes you think you can do better?"

But as Roy's health and spirit spiraled, Laurentine and I continued to look for answers. In early 2003 we found ourselves attending a Tony Robbins seminar. Tony is an internationally renowned peak-performance and motivational expert. His talk that day opened our eyes. Discussing the importance of nutrition, Tony talked about greens, alkalizing, detoxification, and the dangers of modern processed foods, conventional fruits and vegetables laden with pesticides, and factory-farmed meat and dairy. We knew a little about health and nutrition, but Tony's talk inspired a new desire to discover the facts about health and wellness. We grabbed every book we could find and started researching.

We soon learned that healthy food could be used to heal. We also discovered that the healthcare, food, and agricultural industries were not particularly concerned about our health. They were primarily interested in profits. For example, we learned that the processing of many of our basic foods was not for any health or nutritional benefit. Instead, it was introduced as a way to increase the shelf life and marketability of the industries' products.

We couldn't believe what we uncovered. Our new discoveries convinced us to formalize our knowledge through the Global College of Natural Medicine's Nutritional Consultant program. After completing our studies, we felt even more confident that we could help Roy.

We started sending him some of the books we had been studying. Unfortunately, this seemed to have very little impact. Getting him motivated to read three hundred pages on natural healing remedies was like trying to make water flow uphill. We needed a better way.

FOOD MATTERS: You Are What You Eat

This is how Laurentine and I came up with FOOD MATTERS. If we couldn't get my father to read about nutrition and natural health, we figured we could probably convince him to watch a film on the subject.

We had researched many of the films that existed on the topic. Although many were good and some were excellent, we weren't convinced that any of these films would win over my father. Let's face it, the alternative health industry has a bit of a bad reputation. When most people picture a natural therapist, they envision a man or a woman in sweatpants or a dashiki spinning crystals in his or her backyard. They certainly don't picture a doctor who can help them get better. And Roy was no different. We knew he needed to see natural health in a new light. So we decided to make a film that would restore the image of the wonderful men and women who, through their life-changing work, live up to Hippocrates's famous saying, "Let thy food be thy medicine and thy medicine be thy food."

We invested our life's savings into making FOOD MATTERS. We bought some film equipment and traveled around the world—from Holland, Laurentine's home country, and England to the East and West Coasts of the United States, and then Australia—to interview all of the doctors, nutritionists, scientists, and wellness experts we had been studying throughout Roy's illness.

After our second month of filming, we brought the raw footage to Roy, telling him we weren't leaving until he got well. We were on a mission, and no one could stop us—not even Roy or his team of doctors. As a family, we watched the unedited interviews. Before long, Roy was hooked. What stood out, he told us later, was the story about one of his many medications and how it often caused suicidal thoughts. This was Roy's worst fear. He couldn't believe the pharmaceutical and medical industries would knowingly produce and sell a product that could potentially cause people to physically harm themselves. Not only was modern medicine's better-living-through-chemistry approach not helping, it was making him worse. Almost immediately, he went from believing in the medical profession to believing in the age-old adage "You are what you eat."

Together, Laurentine and I conducted what we like to call a "fridge audit." We threw out any food that wasn't real. This included all of the diet products, all of the processed foods and fats, and all of the factory-farmed meat and dairy. We then guided Roy through a detoxification program, adding in more and more healthy foods to his diet. At the same time, we helped wean him off his medications by putting him on a special—and closely monitored—natural supplement regimen. Roy agreed to our help against the wishes of his team of doctors. They tried to scare him and pushed for more medications. When he told them he wanted to stop, the doctors responded with horror stories about what would happen if he did, including all of the potential symptoms associated with withdrawal.

Within a few months, Roy was back to his old self. Maybe even better. He was out of bed, moving freely and energetically around the house. He lost weight and was no longer anxious or depressed. He slept through the night and woke up each morning refreshed and ready for the day. He even started jogging again, something he hadn't done in years. He was renewed. A simple commitment to natural foods freed him from the chronic fatigue syndrome that had trapped him for over five years. It was amazing to watch.

Laurentine and I knew we had to show our documentary to as many people as possible and explain where the food, agricultural, and pharmaceutical industries have gone wrong, while offering the audience natural solutions to everyday health problems. Since its release in May 2008, *FOOD MATTERS* has been seen by millions of people online, in theaters, on television, on airlines, and even in hospitals and community centers around the world, from Connecticut to Cambodia, in nine different languages.

HUNGRY FOR CHANGE:
Your Health Is in Your Hands

What struck us most about Roy's recovery was the reaction from his friends and family. At family gatherings and events, the first thing they would say to Roy was "Wow, you look amazing! Your skin is vibrant, you've lost so much weight, and you even look younger! What have you been doing?" They had little interest in hearing about how he kicked his medications and conquered his illness. They only cared about his physical appearance and how they too could lose weight, improve their appearance, and regain more energy. At this point we knew that we had another film on our hands and that it had the potential to reach an even wider audience.

We discovered there were so many people who have tried—and failed—to lose weight through the latest fad diets or weight-loss products. All too many people, we realized, deal with excess weight, bloating, acid reflux, skin irritations, food cravings, emotional eating, high blood pressure, and an addiction to processed and sugary foods. All of these are signs that the body is out of balance. Many turn to diets and diet products and become slaves to an endless cycle: what we call the diet trap. But the good news is that a total health transformation is possible through a natural diet of fresh, delicious, and wonderful foods packed with life-sustaining nutrients.

HUNGRY for CHANGE is dedicated to helping people escape the diet trap. The food industry has led us to believe that its products are going to make us healthy, happy, sexy, and young. These promises are as empty as the food and drinks they're trying to sell us. The truth is we've never been fatter or in worse health. *HUNGRY for CHANGE* reveals the diet, weight-loss, and food industries' deceptive and manipulating strategies that keep us coming back for more, even when we know we shouldn't.

We wanted to show people that the only way to achieve the body and health we all want and deserve is through a natural diet. But we couldn't do this on our own. Just as we did for *FOOD MATTERS*, we enlisted the help of the world's leading natural health and medical experts, and men and women who discovered lasting weight loss, abundant energy, and vibrant health after years of being sick and overweight. Their stories prove that it's possible to break free from years of bad eating habits and start on a journey to better health.

We invite you to join us and take control of your health and your life. Your health is in your hands.

Part I

HUNGRY FOR CHANGE

CHAPTER ONE

How Did We Get Here?

T hroughout history, humans have struggled to find calories. Thousands of years ago, when we lived outdoors, we didn't always know when or where we'd find our next meal. Our bodies held on to extra weight in order to protect us from famines. This is because when our hunter-gatherer-gardener ancestors—and this goes right up to a few hundred years ago—found sources of fat or sugar, it meant survival. It meant they could carry forth their genetic line.

"It's not your fault," says Christiane Northrup, M.D., a bestselling author and an expert on women's health. "You're programmed to put on fat whenever there is food available. This is how we are as mammals. We've lived on the earth for millennia where there was a food shortage. But now there is a lot of food available, but it's the wrong kind. And so we've been programmed for millennia to store up for the winter, but the winter doesn't come."

The human body comes with ready-made fat programs, according to Jon Gabriel, a weight-loss expert and international bestselling author of *The Gabriel Method*, because these programs protect us against famines. "The human body," he says, "evolved to survive during a famine or a cold winter or whatever kind of stress. What this means is your body is designed to hold extra weight during a period of stress, and if you go through a stress today, your body will hold on to an extra 10 pounds to protect itself."

Because our bodies are biologically adapted to store fat, we continue to seek out calories, particularly fats and sugars. If we taste something fatty, for instance, or something sweet, the body sends us an immediate signal that says, "Yes, I want more of this." Craving these foods is perfectly normal. So when we bite into a burger or take a sip of a milk shake, and we taste those fats and those sugars again, our bodies tell us to eat, because they are used to living in an environment where there is feast and famine. "The problem today," says Daniel Vitalis, a leading health, nutrition, and personal development strategist, "is we've got feast like nobody's business. We just don't have any famine. We have an almost unlimited supply of calorie sources. And this is where we run into problems. We're eating too much of the wrong foods."

If we look around the world, we see that human beings have been able to inhabit the whole globe. They've been able to do it on a host of different foods—from the extreme Arctic, where people have eaten almost exclusively animal fat and muscle and organ meats, to the jungle, where people had access to far more fruits and plant material.

"One of the things we see in the food of today's hunter-gatherer-gardener people is that it contains an extremely high amount of nutrition and an extremely low amount of calories," says Vitalis. "We see people thriving and people staying lean and healthy and avoiding degenerative diseases and not putting on extra weight, regardless of what or how much they eat. We see people living in harmony with their ecosystems and their bodies."

Today, our diet no longer resembles that. Our so-called modern foods contain a very high number of calories and a very low amount of nutrition. We no longer eat the foods we're biologically adapted to—the simple foods: plant foods, fruits, nuts, seeds, vegetables, and animal foods of high quality. We've gone from living off our natural environ-

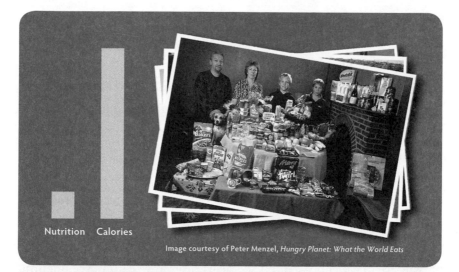

Nutrition Calories

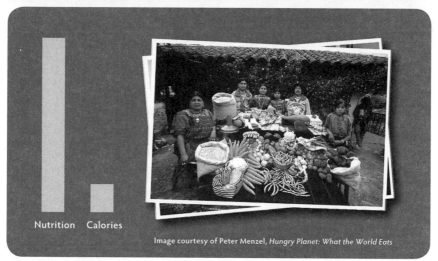

Nutrition Calories

ment as hunter-gatherer-gardener people did—and still do in some places—to eating industrialized, genetically modified, and artificially produced foods. At the same time, we've adopted this relatively new indoor, sedentary lifestyle. Our bodies are not designed to sit at desks under fluorescent lights and eat processed junk food all day long.

By overloading on processed food and ignoring the vitamins, minerals, fibers, and healthy fats that we need, we are essentially poisoning ourselves with calories. We are simultaneously overeating *and* starving ourselves to death. And so we keep eating and keep eating and keep eating, which leads to more and more problems. We see things like diabetes. We see blood sugar imbalance issues, and we see a lot of weight gain.

"This is not the case with indigenous cultures," Vitalis says. "Their diet is typically lower in calories but has ten times the fat-soluble vitamins, like vitamins A, E, D, and K, than our modern diet. And indigenous diets contain four times the water-soluble vitamins—vitamins B and C. There is more nutrition in their food than in our recommended daily allowance of nutrients. We don't see the same chronic, degenerative diseases we see in so-called modern people. We don't see the prevalence of cancer. We don't see heart disease. We don't see arthritic conditions. If we continue to live only on the processed foods we find in our modern supermarkets, we're going to constantly have problems.

"Because these foods make us fat.

"These foods make us sick.

"These foods break down our pancreas and give us diabetes.

"These foods give us cancer."

So, how do we wean ourselves off these foods? Easy. By eating food in its simplest and most wild form. When we step outside of that supermarket setting, when we start going to the farmers' markets, when we start going to the farms, we don't have to worry about these problems anymore. We can let our bodies guide us. We don't have to worry about putting on weight—or keeping it off—because the body doesn't want to be overweight.

Your body is designed to be healthy. It *wants* to be healthy. One of the biggest tricks the marketing industry has used against us is to convince us that our bodies are trying to get fat. And we have to somehow whip them into shape, stop them, fight them all the time. That's simply not true.

If we let our body do what it wants to do in an environment full of healthy choices, then we can live without fear of weight gain and we can live without fear of degenerative disease.

What's an Unhealthy Diet?

"You are what you eat." It's a saying as old as written history. But before we can even talk about the consequences of unhealthy food choices for a nation, we have to engage in some honest talk about what is considered an unhealthy diet.

The U.S. Department of Agriculture (USDA) wants Americans to eat more of everything—more dairy, more meat, more grains, and even more sugar. To its mind, "poor nutrition" just means people aren't eating enough dairy, meat, grains, and sugar. The USDA remains stuck in the mindset of the 1930s, when people were literally starving from a lack of calories. So the USDA policy incessantly remains, "Eat more!"

But Americans don't need to eat more. They need to eat less. A lot less. And especially less of the highly toxic, disease-promoting foods described below.

According to Mike Adams, researcher and founder of NaturalNews .com, these are the main characteristics of an unhealthy diet:

- Primarily consists of dead foods (cooked, microwaved, etc.)

- Primarily consists of refined grains (milled, bleached, etc.)

- Lacks large quantities of fresh, living fruits and vegetables

- Avoids adequate water hydration (and focuses on manufactured beverages)

- Is very high in processed sugars and processed carbohydrates

- Contains genetically modified (GM) foods, such as corn and soy, and sugar from GM sugar beets

- Includes a large amount of hormone-laden and pasteurized conventional dairy products, such as cow milk

- Is made with hundreds of different chemical food additives, from MSG and aspartame to chemical preservatives

- Is packaged in toxic containers including plastics and epoxy resins that contaminate the food with bisphenol A (BPA)

- Primarily consists of conventionally grown, pesticide-contaminated foods

- Contains a large quantity of unhealthy oils, such as corn, soy, or partially hydrogenated oils

- Consists of a large number of fried foods or foods cooked at a very high temperature, which destroys nutrients while also creating carcinogenic compounds

- Is made with many modified, unnatural ingredients, such as hydrogenated oils, refined sugars (the refining process removes the minerals), homogenized milk fats, and so on

- Consists of a large quantity of factory-farmed and factory-fed animal products

❯ Profile in Health

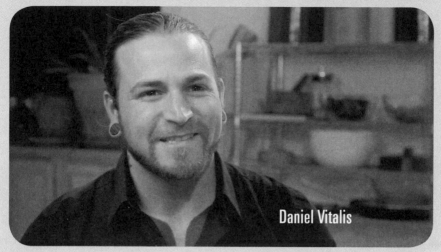

Daniel Vitalis

I grew up in the United States in the 1980s, a red-blooded product of the industrial food complex. I was exposed to all kinds of processed and refined foods. I ate white bread, white flour, processed corn- and soy-based products. I grew up on pasteurized industrial dairy products, and my meat came wrapped in Styrofoam and plastic.

Mostly, though, I ate food that came in different shapes and colors—foods, I understand now, that were more about marketing than nutrition. Boxed cereals were my favorite. When my mother brought me to the supermarket, a big, glitzy, glamorous mall of processed foods, I used to run right to the cereal aisle, begging her for a specific kind of cereal because of the cartoon character on the packaging. I craved it all the time.

Like everyone else in my generation, I grew up in a giant international food experiment. Call us the Genetically Modified Generation. But here's the thing. That experiment failed us.

I had a lot of respiratory issues as a kid. I thought I had asthma. I was hyper-inflamed all the time, and I had no idea it was because of the kinds of food I was eating.

Until I was about fifteen. A friend of mine handed me a copy of The Grape Cure, which basically chronicled a group of people who harvested grapes in Europe for wine. During the process, they fasted on grapes for a couple of weeks. Because of this fast, according to the book, they prevented a lot of the same chronic, degenerative diseases we see today in our culture, particularly cancers. That's when I started to understand the idea that food could be like a medicine for us, and we could use food to cleanse and rejuvenate our bodies. And if we did that periodically, we might even be able to live longer, healthier lives.

Which made me think about the food I was eating. Where did it come from? Why was I eating it? Questions like these made me want to change my diet. And you know what? Once I did, my health problems started to go away. Ever since, I've been on a quest to bring this message to the world.

Throughout my career, I've studied indigenous peoples of the planet. Up until 200 years ago, indigenous people lived in harmony with their ecosystems and their bodies. They didn't have the chronic degenerative diseases we have today. They didn't break down the way we're breaking down today.

We've gone from an organism that lives in environments just as the hunter-gatherer people all over the world did, and still do in some places, to a fully domesticated species that survives on synthetically processed foods and comes in regular contact with different plastics and petrochemicals, which we absorb through our skins—everything from cellophane to a nylon comforter.

We've become strangers to nature. And the best way to live longer, healthier lives is to re-wild ourselves by returning to nature whenever we can. Replace the nylon comforter with a cotton or down one. Replace the GORE-TEX jacket with wool. Replace the plastic couch with natural materials. Add in locally produced flour for white flour. Add in locally produced organic milk for pasteurized and mass-produced milk. Move in a direction that brings you closer toward a re-approximation of your natural diet.

I still eat the same kinds of foods I grew up with. I just eat the real versions of them, the wild versions with all of the goodness and nutrients that keep me lean, trim, vibrant, and healthy.

❯ A nature-based philosopher, Daniel Vitalis is a leading health, nutrition, and personal development strategist. He teaches that our invincible health is a product of living in alignment with our biological design and our role in the ecosystem. He incorporates the wisdom of indigenous peoples into our modern lives. His website is www.danielvitalis.com.

Manufactured Addictions

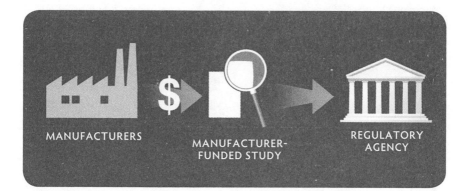

MANUFACTURERS   MANUFACTURER-FUNDED STUDY   REGULATORY AGENCY

One of the biggest causes of obesity is addiction. People simply can't stop eating foods they know are bad for them. We all understand addiction to cigarettes. We all understand addiction to alcohol. But we don't yet fully understand addiction to food, even though the food industry knowingly adds addictive chemicals into our food, not unlike how the tobacco industry knowingly added nicotine to cigarettes in order to make them addictive.

The food industry engineers addictions into many of our foods. It is a multibillion-dollar industry with the scientific resources and the wherewithal to identify what tastes good to the average consumer and then manufacture chemical derivatives of that flavor into our food. Those chemical derivatives often include an addictive component.

"The objective of the food industry is not to give you a product that is healthy," says Alejandro Junger, M.D., bestselling author of *Clean: The Revolutionary Program to Restore the Body's Natural Ability to Heal Itself.* "It is to give you a product that will make you want to buy it, that will have a long shelf life, and that will make a lot of money for the people producing it." The food industry's goal is to sell you more food.

"And what's the best way to do this?" asks addiction specialist and bestselling author Jason Vale. "By manipulating the chemical structure

FAST FOOD, FAT PROFITS

Since 2001, the year-on-year annual revenues of America's fast food industry have increased by about 20 percent. At the same time, the number of fast food ads directed at American children has also increased. According to Eric Schlosser, author of *Fast Food Nation*, the typical preschooler now sees about three fast food ads on television every day, while the typical teenager sees about five. "The endless barrage of ads, toys, contests, and marketing gimmicks fuels not only fast food sales, but also a wide range of diet-related illnesses," he wrote on *The Daily Beast* on the tenth anniversary of the publication of his book. "About two-thirds of the adults in the United States are obese or overweight. The obesity rate among preschoolers has doubled in the past thirty years. The rate among children aged six to eleven has tripled. And by some odd coincidence, the annual cost of the nation's obesity epidemic—about $168 billion, as calculated by researchers at Emory University—is the same as the amount of money Americans spent on fast food in 2011."

of food so it's empty but tastes like it's the best and most fulfilling thing we've ever eaten."

A processed, refined-sugar-based food, for instance, or a soda made with high-fructose corn syrup delivers a biochemical charge to our brains that makes us feel momentarily uplifted or momentarily happy. And we get used to that feeling, which makes us want to slam cookies or fast food or sodas to get more of that momentary feeling of elation. But then that feeling very quickly drops off and we're left unfulfilled. Where are the things that the body and the mind really crave? The answer, according to the food industry, is to buy another can of soda or have another cookie or piece of cake.

We literally can't get enough.

"Highly intelligent people around the world are getting morbidly obese," says Vale. "They know full well that the foods they are consuming will kill them. And that's not just eventually, but on a daily basis. They're dying a very slow death. Why do they keep doing this? Because they can't stop. They're addicted." Vale adds, "It's like being in quicksand and constantly being told to get out, but the nature of the beast is to drag you farther down. Addictions transcend logic and intelligence—luckily there is a way out."

MSG, Aspartame, and Caffeine

At the heart of these addictions are MSG, aspartame, and caffeine.

Monosodium glutamate, more commonly known as MSG, is a processed glutamic acid. MSG is also often labeled as E621, yeast extract, autolyzed yeast, hydrolyzed vegetable protein, or sodium caseinate, among others.

"MSG and free glutamates are used to enhance the flavor in about 80 percent of all processed foods," says Raymond Francis, an MIT-trained scientist and registered nutrition consultant.

It's found in the vast majority of processed foods, dietary supplements, cosmetics, personal care products, pharmaceuticals, and pet food.

"MSG first started to be used in food during wartime [World War II] and added into the sea rations of Japanese soldiers to increase taste and stimulate appetite," according to Russell Blaylock, M.D., a board-certified neurosurgeon and noted author. "They had discovered long ago that if you add a little bit of monosodium glutamate, it makes food

"MSG and free glutamates are used to enhance the flavor in about 80 percent of all processed foods."

—RAYMOND FRANCIS

taste very good. So if you take a very bad tasting food, particularly canned foods, which have that tinny-type taste, and you put MSG in it, it just tastes scrumptious. Well, when the food manufacturers got word of this discovery, they too started adding MSG to food, including baby foods."

In addition to making us want to eat more, MSG actively excites the part of our brains in charge of our fat programs. Once that part of our brains is excited, our bodies activate these programs, which make us hold on to fat. "Every scientist knows this," says Jon Gabriel. "When you want to study obesity and you want to study a fat mouse, you have to make a mouse fat, because mice aren't fat. So the way you make a mouse fat is by feeding him MSG. There's even a term for it. It's called MSG obesity-induced mice. And this is in 80 percent of modern-day foods."

Google it.

Just as MSG wreaks havoc on our brain, so too do aspartame and other artificial sweeteners. These sweeteners include dangerous toxic substances that can wreak havoc on our bodies. Aspartame is most commonly found in many diet and sugar-free varieties of foods and drinks—everything from sodas to breath mints to cookies to cereals to iced teas and juice drinks.

Dr. Joseph Mercola, an osteopathic physician, wrote a book about artificial sweeteners titled *Sweet Deception*. He says these are far worse for us than sugar. "Aspartame is marketed as natural, but it's actually a dipeptide, which means there are two amino acids linked together, aspartic acid and phenylalanine. Well, those two amino acids are natural, but they were never designed to be linked together like that and then taken in such large amounts. They're actually connected with what's called an ester bond. When this ester bond breaks apart, methanol is transported past the blood–brain barrier and goes into the brain and turns to formaldehyde, which is very, very toxic and could cause tumors, seizures, migraines, and headaches."

ASPARTAME

James Schlatter, a chemist at G.D. Searle and Company, discovered aspartame in 1965 while researching an anti-ulcer drug. It was approved for use in dry goods in 1981 and approved for use in carbonated beverages two years later, in 1983. Aspartame—marketed under the brand names NutraSweet, Equal, and Canderel—is often listed as E951.

Aspartame can be commonly found in the following foods and drinks:

Breath mints	Juice drinks
Carbonated soft drinks	Maple syrup
Cereal	Nutritional bars
Chewing gum	Slushies
Fat-free yogurts	Sugar-free cookies
Flavored coffee syrups	Sugar-free gelatin
Flavored water	Sugar-free ice cream
Hard candy	Table sweeteners
Iced tea	Vegetable drinks

Other ailments include neurological and cognitive problems that often mimic multiple sclerosis.

"Nothing else does it in your brain quite like a diet soda," says Dr. Northrup. "And that's because there's a deadly combination of aspartame and caffeine. Those two together create a very unique blend of excitotoxin that kills off brain cells. But before they die they have this excitement that's like a buzz. So what you find with brand-name diet soda addicts, particularly women who want to keep their weight down, is they sometimes drink a liter to two liters a day. They don't eat. They just have the next buzz of diet soda. Over time, this can lead to symptoms that mimic multiple sclerosis. There's headaches. There's neurologic problems. There's all kinds of problems."

Sugar Is a Drug

The number one source of calories in the United States is fructose, and it's highly addictive.

"When it comes to high-fructose corn syrup," says Mike Adams, a consumer health advocate and editor of NaturalNews.com, "a lot of people don't realize its dangers. High-fructose corn syrup obviously comes from corn, but it's not natural, because it's an isolated nutrient. For example, cocaine comes from coca leaves, and coca leaf tea is perfectly safe for your health. There's no harm in drinking coca tea, and it's not addictive, but you wouldn't want to snort cocaine from the highly refined coca tea.

"Well, eating high-fructose corn syrup, in my opinion, is a lot like snorting cocaine. It is the highly refined, isolated and concentrated, chemically manipulated version of something that's found and grown in corn."

Which helps explain why we're hooked on fructose and why our addiction to it is getting worse. In the 1900s, the average person consumed about 15 grams of fructose, or less than an ounce a day. The average person today consumes 70 to 80 grams a day, and there are many kids, primarily teenagers, who are taking in 120, 130, or 150 grams of fructose a day. That's literally ten times the amount people ingested a century ago.

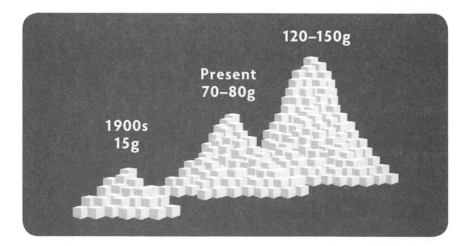

This type of exposure can lead to some very severe metabolic consequences and exacerbate addictive processes, which make it next to impossible to break the cycle of craving unhealthy foods and drinks.

In terms of just the glycemic index (an indication of how quickly foods convert into sugar in the blood), high-fructose corn syrup is like jet fuel for your body. If you pour jet fuel into your car's gasoline tank, you're going to ruin your engine and burn it out. Much the same thing happens in the human body.

While there's nothing entirely wrong with a little sugar now and again, it's crucial to define what we mean by moderation, because we seem to have lost the basic concept of moderation. Americans today consume about 150 pounds of sugar and 79 pounds of high-fructose corn syrup per year. That amounts to about 22 teaspoons of sugar per day.

Sugar is in everything—from cough syrup to crackers to cereal to sushi. It's almost impossible to avoid. But here comes the tricky part: When you're thinking about what to eat, if you're working to reduce your sugar intake, your definition of what sugar is really needs to expand.

There are many different forms of sugar—white crystallized sugar, maple syrup, malted barley, fruit sugar, and high-fructose corn syrup, but even processed carbohydrates are a form of sugar. Once your body breaks down these carbohydrates, they turn to sugar, immediately increasing sugar levels in your bloodstream. "Most things contain sugar or are, in fact, sugar," says Jason Vale. "You think of something like a croissant. People say, 'I've gone on a sugar-free diet,' but they're eating a croissant. And I say that's sugar. What do you think is going to happen when that enters the bloodstream? That is sugar."

So it's more than just the white crystals. It's bread, pasta, cereal, rice, potatoes, corn, waffles, pancakes, and pretty much any food most Americans eat for breakfast.

When we're depressed or under stress, we crave foods that make us feel good, comfort foods like macaroni and cheese, which give us that sugar high. We become addicted to that high, just as we do with other drugs, and we need more and more and more over time to give us that same effect.

"It's not fat that makes us fat," says Dr. Northrup, "it's sugar that makes us fat." The more sugar we consume, the more we experience chronic disease, as well as these incredible up and down mood swings. This is because sugar increases beta-endorphins in the brain, the feel-good, natural opiate, morphine-like substance.

We normally associate addiction with cocaine, heroin, and other big drugs, but the truth is that more premature deaths are the result of sugar and alcohol and smoking than cocaine or heroin.

"If you walk the aisles in the average grocery store and look at the amount of sugar in a child's breakfast cereal," says Dr. Northrup, "you might as well be rolling up the kid's sleeve and putting in heroin. Because it's the same. It's that addictive."

We know the problems caused by cocaine and heroin and alcohol. We now regularly refer to them as drugs. It's time we started recognizing white sugar as a drug. To get a handle on our addiction to sugar, we need to start thinking about these massive doses of sugar as no different from drugs and alcohol.

Healthy Sweetener Comparison Chart

LESS HEALTHY

Artificial sweeteners, including aspartame

High-fructose corn syrup

White refined sugar

Agave nectar

Raw cane sugar

Coconut palm sugar

Raw unprocessed honey or maple syrup

Dates, raisins, or fresh fruit used in juices or smoothies

MORE HEALTHY — Stevia (natural herb sweetener)

Profile in Health

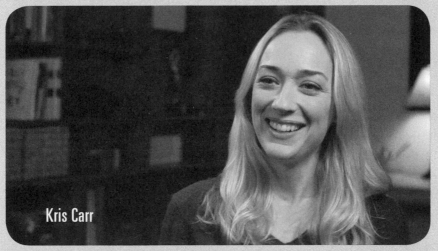

Kris Carr

O n Valentine's Day 2003, I was diagnosed with a rare and incurable stage four cancer. In an instant, I went from hot chick to sick chick, saddled with an extremely rare sarcoma called epithelioid hemangioendothelioma (EHE), which affects less than 0.01 percent of the cancer population. Little is known about my annoyingly hard-to-spell-and-pronounce disease, and none of the "Big C" cancer bucks go into studying it. The cancer, I quickly found out, was inoperable—no surgery, radiation, chemotherapy—and here's the knockout punch: no cure!

Fortunately, my cancer was slow moving and essentially chronic, which gave me what all cancer patients want: time. Rather than taking a wait-and-see approach, however, I decided to take a watch-and-live approach and do everything in my power to make sure my cancer didn't make the first move.

Step one was to learn how to take care of myself. I was thirty-one, and I didn't know how to feed myself. I had to stop everything and go back and learn all of the things I wish I had known as a child, as a teenager, as a young adult.

My wake-up moment sparked in me a deep desire to stop holding back and start living like I mean it! If I couldn't be cured, I wondered, could I still be healthy? And if so, maybe, just maybe I could help my body and my mind keep the disease in check.

I made a total lifestyle upgrade inside and out. I learned how to listen to my brilliant internal guide, which brought me back to nature (my church), the garden, and the people and animals who set my heart ablaze. I learned that a nutrient-dense, plant-based diet rules, the Standard American Diet kills, stress sucks (all life force), exercise is non-negotiable, joy is utterly contagious, and having fun must be taken seriously.

❯ Kris Carr is the *New York Times* bestselling author of *Crazy Sexy Diet, Crazy Sexy Cancer Tips, Crazy Sexy Cancer Survivor,* and *Crazy Sexy Kitchen.* A motivational speaker and wellness coach, she leads workshops at wellness centers throughout the United States and lectures at medical schools, hospitals, and universities. Kris has been featured on *The Today Show, Good Morning America, The CBS Evening News, The Gayle King Show,* and *The Oprah Winfrey Show.* She is the founder of the award-winning online magazine *Crazy Sexy Life* at crazysexylife.com.

CHAPTER TWO

The Diet Trap

According to the January 20, 2010, issue of *Journal of the American Medical Association*, 68 percent of adults in the United States are overweight or obese. That's an astounding number. It's the kind of number that makes us want to do whatever it takes to lower it.

"America loves enemies," says Alejandro Junger, M.D., author of the *New York Times* bestseller *Clean*. "America chooses an enemy and employs all of its forces against it. At some point, when we noticed we were getting fat, we made fat the enemy and attacked it. Everything became fat-free. And we replaced fat with carbohydrates. As a result, we became the fattest country in the world."

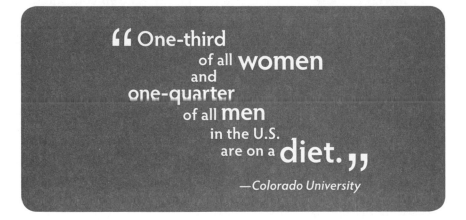

❝ One-third of all **women** and **one-quarter** of all **men** in the U.S. are on a **diet. ❞**
—*Colorado University*

Here's the thing about fat-free. It's a farce. Fat-free food just means it's loaded with sugar. "I can get a two-pound bag of sugar and put a label [on it] that says it's 100 percent fat-free," says Jason Vale, bestselling author of *7 Lbs in 7 Days* and founder of Juice Master. "While factually correct, it's also incredibly misleading. Once a person ingests that sugar, the pancreas immediately secretes insulin—a fat-producing hormone—to lower the rise in the body's sugar levels.

"So all this excess energy comes along, and the body has to store it somewhere. In the short term, the body stores it in the liver. But to store the excess energy, the body produces fat cells, thinking it can just burn them off later. The problem is, with a fat-free diet, there's never a later."

When you're on a fat-free or low-fat diet, you're constantly hungry. Why? Because your body needs the correct fats and proteins to function. If you cut out either of those, your body will cry out for them.

We've been tricked into believing a fat-free or sugar-free diet is healthy. It's not. A lot of these products contain very questionable, possibly toxic ingredients that are incredibly bad for you.

The business of marketing food and beverages is the business of getting people to make purchasing decisions that are not in their best long-term interest. Many of these foods promote heart disease, diabetes, and cancer, but marketers want you to think that it's in your interest somehow to keep buying that product.

Fats are actually really good for you. The key is eating the right kinds of fats. Cheap, low-grade fats, such as soybean oil, canola oil, and corn oil, are bad fats and extremely unhealthy in large quantities. Partially hydrogenated fats are even worse. These are used in many commercially baked items, crackers, cookies, and margarine spreads—some of the worse foods you could possibly eat. Healthy fats are usually found in natural plant- and animal-based foods, such as avocados, chia seeds and flaxseeds, or wild-caught fish, like salmon or trout.

Food Advertising and Labeling

The good news is, more and more people are wising up to the fat-free farce, despite the food industry's best efforts. Look at the way they market soda. They present you with an image of a can of soda, but they never tell you what's in the can. They only tell you that if you drink it, you'll be cool, or sexy, or happy and surrounded by beautiful, happy people.

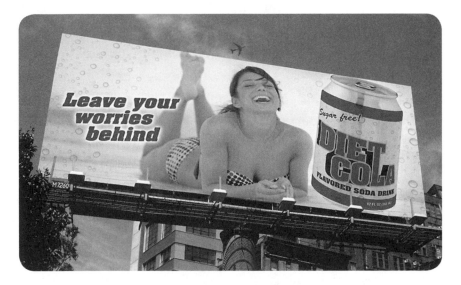

But if you drink that can of soda, you'll likely lose bone mineral density because of the phosphoric acid it contains. If it's a diet soda, it contains chemical sweeteners, which can lead to neurological problems, and if it's not a diet soda, it likely contains high-fructose corn syrup (in North America, at least), which promotes type 2 diabetes and obesity. Plus, studies show that if you drink diet soda, it increases carbohydrate cravings, which often leads to even more weight gain.

The food industry promises you one thing and delivers another.

This deception isn't limited to their marketing and advertising campaigns, according to Mike Adams, editor of NaturalNews.com.

Food labels are also deceptive. "The way major food companies name their food products," he says, "is a little too loose and creative. It's almost as if they're naming them based on what they hope you might imagine you're eating rather than what's really in the box, because there's a whole lot of stuff in there they don't want you to read on the label. Stuff like propylene glycol, a chemical used in a lot of blueberry muffins and blueberry-flavored cereals. It's used to make up the blueberry bits that aren't actually blueberries. They are made out of propylene glycol, partially hydrogenated oils, liquid sugars, and artificial colors.

"Well, you can also use propylene glycol to winterize your RV, because it keeps your pipes from freezing in the winter. It's also used to clean out your colon before a colonoscopy."

When you're reading food labels, make sure you read the list of ingredients. Watch out for artificial food colors, anything with a number and color, like FFDC Red Number 40 (E129) or Blue Number 2 (E132). A general rule of thumb, as articulated by Michael Pollan in *Food Rules: An Eaters Manual:* If your grandmother wouldn't recognize it as food, don't eat it.

Look out for yeast extract or torula yeast, which is just another form of MSG. These contain free glutamic acid, a highly addictive excitotoxin.

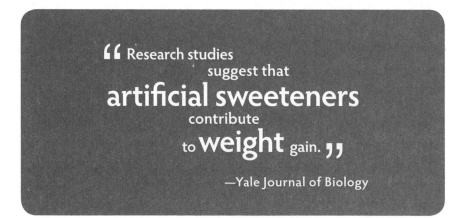

" Research studies suggest that **artificial sweeteners** contribute to **weight** gain. "

—Yale Journal of Biology

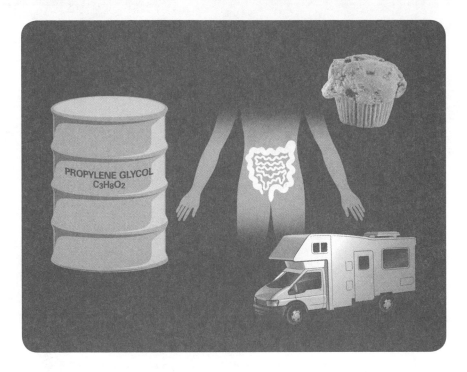

Watch out especially for sugar-free labels. Just because it says sugar-free, doesn't mean it's healthy. Sugar-free foods often contain chemical sweeteners, such as aspartame, acesulfame potassium (Acesulfame K), sucralose, or saccharin, which can also be found in children's cough medicines and chewable vitamins.

› Profile in Health

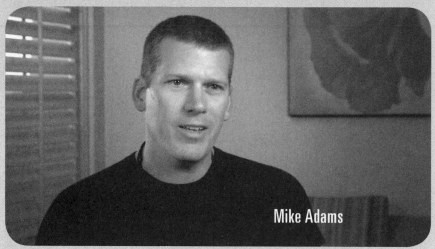

Mike Adams

The only thing that stands between you and your own perfect health is information. Empowered with the right information, you can improve your health, reduce your dependence on prescription drugs, enhance your quality of life, and expand your mental awareness and creativity.

It's not complicated. The human body already knows how to be healthy. All you have to do is give your body the nutrition it needs so it has the right building materials in place to heal disease and rebuild itself from the inside out.

Today, more than 95 percent of all chronic disease is caused by poor food choices, toxic food ingredients, nutritional deficiencies, and a lack of physical exercise. Which means you can prevent almost every kind of chronic disease, in large part, by avoiding certain types of food. Again, it's not complicated.

When I was thirty, I was borderline obese. I was diabetic, and I suffered from chronic pain and depression. I had a lot of health problems. I was miserable. I decided that wasn't the way I wanted to live. I wanted to be healthy. So I started studying. As I read more and more books, I learned more and more about nutrition, which helped me change my diet and my lifestyle. I got rid of sugar. I got rid of cheese and dairy. I got rid of meats (though I now eat some fish).

The changes started to happen automatically. Within six months, I lost 50 pounds. That's the beautiful thing about the human body and its ability to heal itself. If you do the right things, the body will heal itself while you sleep, and you can't even help but heal yourself if you follow the right steps and get in tune with nature.

That's what I did, and that's what I now hope to keep teaching others to do.

A nice trick I tell people is, if you want to eat healthy, eat the foods that are never marketed. Have you ever seen a head of cabbage advertised or marketed? Of course not. But it's one of the best things you could possibly eat. That's true for fresh produce, fresh fruits, roots, nuts, seeds, and healthy fats. Those are the kinds of foods that will make you healthy, and those are the types of foods that are rarely, if ever, promoted.

> Mike Adams, the Health Ranger, is a consumer health advocate and editor of NaturalNews.com.

Why Diets Don't Work

Many of us go on diets to look better. We try different types of fad diets to lose weight in time for swimsuit season, a wedding, or a special occasion. We want to lose weight, and we want to lose weight fast, and in America we're willing to pay for it to the tune of $60 billion a year spent on diet and diet-related products.

"I think we are barking up the wrong tree," says Dr. Junger. "People are looking for a result that is superficial. They want to look good, and they don't really consider that that could be done from the inside out. So people go into diets and all these fads in order to lose weight and lose weight fast, and that is just not the way to approach it. The results prove it."

We can lose weight on a diet, but it's a little bit like borrowing from Peter to pay Paul. We can drop 10 pounds through sheer willpower, but we'll have to pay it back. And pay it back with interest. "Every time we force ourselves to lose weight, our bodies will hold on to extra weight to protect itself from a perceived famine," says Jon Gabriel, who lost more than 220 pounds without dieting or surgery. "Lose 10 pounds, gain 15. How many times has this happened to you? You know people think that overweight people are just weak and lazy and overindulgent.

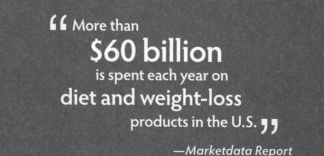

More than
$60 billion
is spent each year on
diet and weight-loss
products in the U.S.

—*Marketdata Report*

> *I want that but I CAN'T have it.*
>
> # I CAN have it
> # but I don't want it.

I am a very disciplined person, but I could not lose the weight when my body wanted to be fat. And neither can you in the short term or the long term. Until you address the real issues."

The entire diet paradigm is flawed. "When people diet, all they're doing is restricting calories or manipulating the way their metabolism works," says David Vitalis, a leading health, nutrition, and personal development strategist. "They can manipulate the ratio of fat to protein to carbohydrate infinitely. There are all these variations. I remember the high-carbohydrate, low-fat diet, then the high-protein, low-carbohydrate, then the low-fat, moderate carbohydrate—it's endless." It seems a new diet comes out every week based on the idea that you can somehow force yourself to lose weight. But that violates our bodies' basic laws of survival.

"I've been on so many diets," says Jason Vale, "and I would immediately start to feel deprived. Think about that. If I weren't on a diet, I could have gone sometimes to two o' clock in the afternoon without thinking about food or even consuming any food. I never thought about it. But the very second I told my brain that I was on a diet, I went into the mode of can't. What I mean by can't is this: CANT, constant and never-ending tantrum. That's all it is, a tantrum. And it's constant and never-ending.

"Now if you go from 'I want that but I can't have it' to 'I can have it but I don't want it,' there's a massive paradigm shift."

Adding In

The best strategy we have for losing weight, according to David Wolfe, nutritionist and superfoods and natural beauty expert, is to add in the good stuff. "Don't turn it into a diet," he says. "If you struggle with dieting, don't eliminate anything from the start. Keep the focus always on adding. Add in the good foods. Add in the foods that aren't man-made, because our bodies don't know how to process these types of foods, which causes us to gain weight. Add in the cucumbers. Add in the apples. Add in the simple foods, the plant-based foods, the fruits, nuts, seeds, vegetables, and the animal products of high quality.

"Eventually the right types of foods will crowd out all the bad stuff. And that works for everybody. It makes everything so simple. It completely deactivates all the mental neuroses we have about diets and what we have to eat. Inevitably, you will start to feel so much better eating the good stuff you won't want to touch the bad stuff."

> Profile in Health

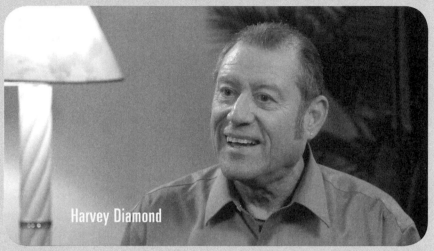

Harvey Diamond

The first chapter of the first book I ever wrote was called "Diets Don't Work." That's because diets have failure built right into them. When people go on a diet, they eliminate protein, fat, or carbohydrates—things we need to live—to shed weight quickly. It works, but once they start eating protein, fat, or carbohydrates again, they put the weight back on immediately. The weight loss is only temporary. Well, let me ask you something: Do you want to be rich temporarily? Of course not. So why would you want to lose weight temporarily?

" Up to two-thirds of those on a diet regain more weight than when they started. "

—University of California, Los Angeles

A study at UCLA once found that up to two-thirds of the people who go on a diet not only gain that weight back, they gain more weight than when they first started. This is because they are so happy to be eating again, they don't eat intelligently.

Which is why, from the very beginning, I've tried to tell people—through my Fit for Life books—to forget about the idea of dieting. Give the body what it needs to take care of itself. We're not designed to be overweight. We weren't put on earth to suffer with every imaginable ache and pain just to counteract our eating habits, because we are doing something that's perfectly normal and natural and necessary to life.

Make your lifestyle such that you eat in a way that your body will automatically maintain a proper body weight for you.

❯ A health and wellness advocate and *New York Times* bestselling author, Harvey Diamond is a pioneer in helping shift people toward healthier eating. Throughout his forty-year career he has helped millions of people around the world improve their health and overcome serious diseases, including cancer. His Fit for Life books have sold nearly 14 million copies and have been translated into 33 different languages. His website is harveydiamond.com.

Part II

YOUR HEALTH IS IN YOUR HANDS

CHAPTER THREE

You Are What You Eat

I f the body is an engine, then food is its fuel. Food gives the body the energy it needs to function. If we don't make sure the fuel we pump through our systems is the right quality and quantity, we're going to run ourselves right onto the scrap heap. The foods we eat affect our weight, mood, energy level, brain function, sex drive, and sleeping patterns.

Healthy eating is essential to our well-being. As discussed in the previous chapter, the best strategy we have for losing weight is to add into our diet the right kinds of foods. The trick is to replace all the manufactured foods we normally eat on a day-to-day basis with local, fresh, organic, and more natural options.

"For me it's back to nature and it's back to the garden," says Kris Carr, author of *Crazy Sexy Diet*. "If it's made in the garden, then I eat it. If it's made in a lab, it takes a lab to digest. If it has a shelf life longer than me, I don't eat it. The simpler I get, the healthier I get."

"The simpler I get, the healthier I get."
—KRIS CARR

Every nutritionist recommends six to eight servings of fruits and vegetables a day. Vegetables, in particular, contain a full range of fiber, nutrients, and anti-oxidants—exactly the kinds of fuel our bodies need to stay healthy.

Mike Adams, the Health Ranger, suggests asking yourself three questions before eating:

Where does my food come from? What went into making the food, in terms of attitude or care or love or compassion? And is this food for nourishment or simply for entertainment? "A lot of people look at food as entertainment, as if their tongue were an amusement park," he says. "They just want the taste sensations—MSG, salt, spices, whatever. And then they swallow it and forget about it. But that food stays in you for a very long time. You should eat food for what it does all the way through your system, not just what it's doing in your mouth. If you want to be healthy, don't treat your mouth like an amusement park."

Top 10 Nutritional Tips

Here are ten handy nutritional tips to ensure your body gets the proper nutrients it needs to function effectively on a daily basis.

❶ Eat as Nature Intended

Nature didn't create you to eat ready-made frozen meals with artificial preservatives and chemicals. Our ancestors have always lived in symbiosis with nature, and humankind has always been geared toward natural food. It's simple: eat more "living" food and eat less "dead" food. This means plenty of fresh vegetables and fruits (in season and in a wide range of colors), herbs, seaweeds, mushrooms, sprouted nuts and seeds, natural yogurt, and cultured vegetables, and if you eat meat and animal products this would also include organic free-range eggs, wild-caught fish, game, and naturally reared animals.

❷ Choose Organic

Organic fruits and vegetables can often contain more vitamins and minerals than their non-organic or conventional counterparts, particularly if they have been picked ripe and are locally grown. They are also safer to eat because they are grown without the use of chemical fertilizers, pesticides, and genetically modified organisms (GMOs), all of which have been shown to have harmful effects on our reproductive health and hormones and overload the liver. If you eat animal products, choose natural dairy from pasture-raised cows, organic free-range eggs, and naturally reared grass-fed or wild meats. It is especially important with animal products to ensure they are free from antibiotics, hormones, and GMO feed, as animal fats tend to concentrate toxins. (See page 260 for the Dirty Dozen and Clean Fifteen lists.)

❸ Dust Off Your Juicer or Blender

A juicer and/or blender can be your best friend. Let's say you come home from work and you're hungry and lethargic. Instead of reaching for a bag of chips or a bar of chocolate, whip up a quick juice or smoothie, both of which are loaded with vitamins, minerals, and enzymes. It's an instant meal that delivers nutrients directly to the cells of your body.

❹ Limit Gluten-Containing Grains

Gluten is a protein found in most grains, including wheat, rye, barley, and spelt. An allergy to gluten—known as coeliac (or celiac) disease—and a general intolerance to gluten are becoming more prevalent. Even if you're not sensitive to gluten, you can do your body a world of good by cutting back on your gluten intake. Gluten can irritate and damage the intestinal lining and cause inflammation or immune reactions. It is also a major cause of leaky gut. Traditional preparation of these grains—soaking them for at least twelve hours and fermenting or sourdough leavening—helps to remove some of the gluten, rendering them less harmful. Great gluten-free grain alternatives include buckwheat, quinoa, rice, millet, corn, and amaranth.

❺ Stay Away from Processed Sugary Foods

Too much sugar or other refined carbohydrates can lead to blood sugar highs and lows, causing mood swings and food cravings, if not balanced by fats and proteins. Opt for foods that naturally have a lower glycemic load or glycemic index (GI). Choose vegetables and low-sugar fruits, such as grapefruits, lemons, limes, pears, berries, and avocados, over starchy grains. If you're going to eat high-GI foods, it's best to combine them with healthy fats to steady the uptake of glucose into the bloodstream. Avoid sweetened packaged foods, particularly those sweetened with high-fructose corn syrup, glucose syrup, or artificial sweeteners.

❻ Eat Good Fats

People trying to lose weight often try to keep their fat and cholesterol intake to a minimum. This is because fat contains more calories per gram than carbohydrates and proteins. Good fats and cholesterol, however, are essential for the absorption of most nutrients and for hormone production. Enjoy the healthy and stable saturated fats found in coconut oil; wild-caught fish; and organic dairy, eggs, and grass-fed meats, as well as monounsaturated fats like extra-virgin olive oil, macadamia nuts, and avocados. Reduce your intake of unstable polyunsaturated fats, such as canola, soy, sunflower, cottonseed, corn, grapeseed, and safflower oils. These oils are often generally labeled as "vegetable oil" and found in products like margarine spreads, commercially baked cookies and potato chips, store-bought mayonnaise and salad dressings, and deep-fried foods.

❼ Prepare Your Meals with Care

Ditch the microwave. Eat more raw foods that have not been damaged by heat. When cooking, sauté, steam, or grill foods over low or medium heat with stable fats, such as coconut oil, ghee, or butter, in an old-fashioned cast-iron pot. These stable saturated fats are less volatile and ideal for cooking, especially compared to most unstable polyunsaturated vegetable oils, which become toxic to the body when oxidized at high temperatures.

❽ Start with a Green Salad

Before your main meal of the day, whether it be lunch or dinner (or both), start with a big green leafy salad. Ditch the iceberg. Be adventurous—choose from romaine, arugula, cabbage, and kale and add chopped mixed fresh herbs like mint, parsley, cilantro, dill, or chives. When you start with a salad, you fill your stomach with nutrient-rich plant foods, leaving less room for overindulging in your entrée or dessert.

❾ Read Labels

Chemical food additives can wreak havoc on our hormones and lead to weight gain and addiction. Avoid E numbers and watch out for MSG, the flavor enhancer that tricks our brains into thinking we need to overeat. MSG is often disguised by the following names: E621, monosodium glutamate, glutamic acid, hydrolyzed vegetable oil, yeast extract, autolyzed yeast, sodium caseinate, and monocalcium glutamate. It is also commonly found in ready-made soups, potato chips, sauces, and cookies. When in doubt, remember one simple tip: If you can't pronounce it, or if it includes numbers or codes, don't eat it!

⑩ Eat in a Relaxed State

Our digestive systems are very sensitive. Rushing through your meal or eating on the run will put your body in a state of fight or flight, which compromises or shuts down your digestive processes, cutting off the assimilation of nutrients into your system. What we don't digest often turns into bacterial fermentation, bloating, or fat. Make sure you are seated and take the time to enjoy your meal in a relaxed state and with good intention.

Know Where Your Food Comes From

Knowing where your food comes from is an important step in improving your nutrition. Speaking with farmers at your local farmers' market and checking the origin of the foods in the produce section of your supermarket will let you know if the food is local or shipped in from far away. Generally speaking, the more local and in-season your food is, the better it is for your health, the environment, and your local food economy.

Food from a factory is unhealthy and unhappy food. It's often trucked in from thousands of miles away. It likely is genetically modified or contains GMO ingredients. It's been processed, hydrogenated, or homogenized. It's barely food at all. Food from a local organic farmer, on the other hand, is happy and healthy food. It's grown in nutrient-rich soil. It's natural. It's good for you, and it tastes better.

It's also a great deal. "When you buy your food from farmers' markets, or when you buy your food directly from farmers, you can actually save a lot more money," according to Daniel Vitalis. "If you go to the farmers' market, for instance, you are buying directly from the source. You've cut out the middleman. You've cut out the store and the driver."

Healthy Food Comparison Chart

LESS HEALTHY	MORE HEALTHY
Conventional milk	Organic cow or goat milk, Homemade Coconut Milk or Nut Milk (see pages 125 and 126), almond milk, macadamia milk, hemp-seed milk
White bread	Sprouted bread, pumpernickel bread, organic sourdough bread, buckwheat crackers
Margarine	Organic butter, mashed-up avocado, extra-virgin olive oil
Boxed cereal	Buckwheat, quinoa, or oat porridge; sprouted cereals; natural granola
Store-bought mayonnaise	Hummus or mashed-up avocado with apple cider vinegar and mustard
Pasta	Spiralized raw vegetables; quinoa, rice, or buckwheat noodles
Cooking oil spray	Organic butter, coconut oil, ghee
Chips and dips	Activated nuts; flaxseed or buckwheat crackers with pesto, hummus, olive tapenade, guacamole, salsa verde, or organic pâté
Ice cream and cake	Non-dairy coconut ice cream, quinoa or rice pudding, Simple Banana Ice Cream (page 236), or Avocado Chocolate Mousse (page 232)
White sugar	Stevia, raw honey, coconut sugar, pure maple syrup
Table salt	Unrefined sea salt, seaweed flakes, miso, tamari, soy sauce
Coffee	Green tea or herbal teas, such as chamomile, jasmine, nettle, mint, roasted dandelion, chicory root
Soda, pop	Water, freshly squeezed juices, sparkling water with fresh lime and raw apple cider vinegar
Milk shake	Berry Kefir Smoothie (page 137), superfood smoothie, freshly squeezed vegetable juices

Shop Around the Outside

If you can't find what you need at the farmers' market, then your best strategy for shopping at a supermarket is to shop around the outside aisles.

Processed foods are normally concentrated in the middle aisles. The freshest and healthiest foods tend to live on the perimeter. If you purchase food located in this part of the supermarket, you'll likely come away better off.

Many of the foods in the center aisles contain food additives to help ease processing, packaging, and storage. But how do we know what food additives are in that box of macaroni and cheese and why it has such a long shelf life? Check the label. A typical American household spends about 90 percent of its food budget on processed foods and, by doing so, is exposed to a plethora of artificial food additives, many of which can result in dire health consequences.

Probiotics: The Keys to the Kingdom

We are often taught that all bacteria and microbes are bad, but there is such a thing as healthy bacteria. Probiotics are a form of healthy bacteria and are essential to life. The word probiotic literally means "good for life." Probiotics are the good bacteria that live in our guts and help us digest our food and assimilate nutrients.

"People don't know this but there are a lot more other organisms in your body than there are cells," says Daniel Vitalis. "And many live in your digestive tract. In fact, there are about four to ten times more bacteria in your gut than there are human cells in your entire body. It's bacteria that take care of you. They colonize you and protect you from organisms that cause disease."

Bad bacteria harbor infectious disease, pathogens, and germs while good bacteria actively work to promote health. If you are not careful, you can deplete your body of good bacteria through an unhealthy diet or the overuse of antibiotics. Without healthy gut bacteria, your stomach loses its ability to digest food and absorb nutrients. Without proper nutrient absorption, your body will constantly be hungry and cause you to crave more and more food, which can lead to obesity. Probiotics are the missing link and are sometimes overlooked in mainstream nutrition and detoxification programs. They are, however, essential to lasting weight loss and optimum health.

One of the best ways to flood your body with probiotics, and push out unhealthy bacteria, is through eating fermented or cultured foods. "Cultured foods have been around as long as people have harvested food," says Vitalis. "This is because we didn't always have refrigeration, and after a few days, food would begin to ferment and break down. Eventually, humans learned how to create beneficial colonies of organisms in these foods. I'm talking about yogurt. I'm talking about kimchi. I'm talking about sauerkraut. I'm talking about wines and beers made in the old way." Other examples of traditionally fermented foods include raw apple cider vinegar, kombucha tea, pickles, and kefir.

Superfoods

All healthy food is not created equal. Some foods are better for us than others. These vibrant, nutritionally rich foods—appropriately called superfoods—offer tremendous dietary and healing potential. Superfoods are powerful sources of clean protein, vitamins, minerals, enzymes, anti-oxidants, good fats and oils, and other nutrients.

Today, when most of us are overfed and undernourished, superfoods can have an extraordinary benefit to our health. "What I finally figured out," says David Wolfe, bestselling author of *Superfoods* and *Eating for Beauty,* "was that we need to take in denser nutrients with each calorie. We eat so much food high in empty calories. There are no minerals. There are no vitamins. There are no polysaccharides. There's no protein." In contrast, superfoods are low in calories but are extraordinarily rich in nutrients. "This is the golden symbol for living longer, while eating less," says Wolfe. "We want stuff that's packed to the hilt but isn't very caloric. Superfoods and super herbs give us the nutrients we need without loading us up with calories."

The best kinds of superfoods are green superfoods. They contain a higher concentration of easily digestible nutrients, fat-burning compounds, vitamins, minerals, and protein that build lean muscles and tissues, aid digestion, and protect you against disease and illness.

Green superfoods are also rich in chlorophyll, the pigment that gives plants their green color. Once broken down, chlorophyll releases hemoglobin into the bloodstream, which in turn increases the level of oxygen in the blood. Green superfoods include spinach, kale, watercress, lettuce, endive, broccoli sprouts and mustard sprouts, spirulina, wheatgrass, barley grass, and wild blue-green algae.

Another kind of superfood is seaweed, the most nutritionally dense plant on the planet. Believe it or not, seaweeds like nori and kelp contain up to ten times more calcium than milk and up to eight times as much as beef. Seaweeds help convert a wide array of food- and environment-related toxins into salt, which the body can more easily eliminate from its system. But the most remarkable benefit of seaweed is its ability to boost weight loss and eliminate cellulite by stimulating the thyroid gland, which breaks down food before it can be turned into fat.

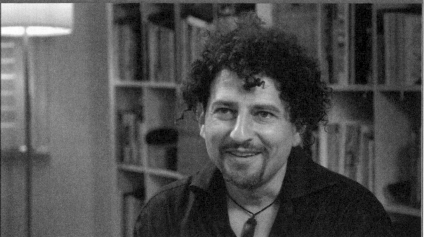

DAVID WOLFE'S TOP 10 SUPERFOODS

Aloe vera

Bee products

Blue-green algae

Cacao (raw chocolate)

Coconuts

Goji berries (Himalayan red berry)

Hemp seed

Maca (Peruvian root)

Marine phytoplankton

Spirulina

❯ David Wolfe is one of the world's leading authorities on nutrition. He is the author of *Eating for Beauty; The Sunfood Diet Success System; Naked Chocolate; David Wolfe on Raw Foods, Superfoods, and Superherbs; Amazing Grace; Superfoods: The Food and Medicine of the Future;* and *The Longevity NOW Program.* His website is www.davidwolfe.com.

CHAPTER FOUR

You Are What You Drink

Juicing

Agreat way to get nutrients directly into your bloodstream is by juicing, especially if you don't like the taste of vegetables. "One of the ways that I cheat this," says Dr. Joseph Mercola, D.O., founder of Mercola.com, "is by doing vegetable juicing. I'll typically buy twenty pounds of vegetables a week and juice a few pounds a day. I like celery and cucumbers as a base and then I add the dark green leafy vegetables like kale or collards."

Juicing gives your body a direct shot of vitamins, minerals, and enzymes. Within a few minutes of downing a glass of liquid nutrition, your body receives an infusion of fuel that nourishes your cells, boosts your metabolism, and helps restore your immune system.

"Juicing is important for two main reasons," according to Jason Vale, a leading expert on health, addiction, and juicing. "People often ask me, 'Why don't you just eat it?' That's a good question. Why don't we just eat it? Well, the answer is we don't eat it. We don't consume enough raw fruits and vegetables in a spectrum of colors. That's number one.

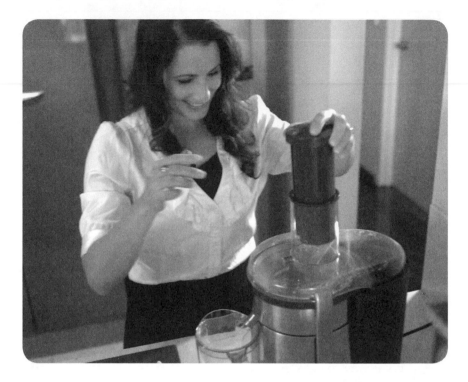

The second thing to remember is most people are overfed and under-nourished. Juicing is important because it's easy to absorb and it's the ultimate fast food. People say, 'I want a fast food diet.' Well, get juicing! Freshly extracted juice is the fifteen-minute nutrient express to health."

Kris Carr, author of *Crazy Sexy Diet*, drinks 16 to 32 ounces of organic green juice every day. "Think about how many cucumbers, kale leaves, and celery stalks I'd have to eat in one sitting to get that many nutrients. It's almost impossible."

> *"Freshly extracted juice is the fifteen-minute*
> *nutrient express to health."*
> —JASON VALE

Her favorite vegetable to juice is cucumber because it's a great source of vitamin C. "These water-filled wonders have a mildly sweet flavor that's easy on the tummy," she says. "Push one or two through your juicer and add whatever other kinds of greens you have, like kale or spinach or romaine, with a little bit of fruit like one green apple and half a peeled lemon, and voilà—you've got a powerful healing elixir! Yummy."

A common mistake made by many newcomers to juicing is to mix in large amounts of fruit, like apples or pears, to sweeten the drink. It's important to limit your body's exposure to sugar, even in the form of fructose. "Fructose is not your friend," says Dr. Mercola. "It is one of the enemies of helping you slow down the aging process. You have to limit fructose, especially in the form of juice. There's nothing wrong with fruit in small quantities, but you have to be careful about raising your fructose levels. Stick to green vegetables."

Dr. Mercola also advises against drinking commercial or manufactured fruit juices. They aren't as healthy as their manufacturers want you to believe. They are pasteurized, or heat processed, for a long shelf life, which results in a loss of vitamins and minerals. They're also fructose-laden and can often contain aspartame.

❯ Profile in Health

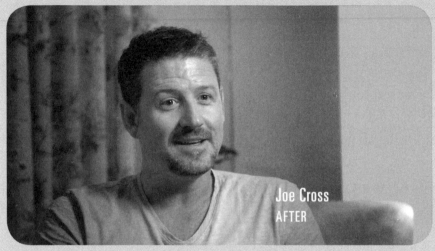

Joe Cross
AFTER

When I was in my early thirties, I focused all of my energy on building my business. My top priority was wealth, and health was way down at the bottom of the list. I was too busy running around the world trying to build my little empire to care about what I did to or put into my body. My diet was poor. I drank too much alcohol. I smoked. I rarely slept. I hardly ever exercised. Eventually, my body gave up. I developed a chronic rash, not unlike hives, which was induced by any kind of touch or pressure on my body. I would swell up all the time. I looked like the Elephant Man. My doctors prescribed for me a powerful steroid called prednisone, which immediately reduced the swelling. One pill and I was healed. I thought, "Wow, isn't it great to be alive in this modern world of medicine?"

But after three or four weeks of taking pills twice a day, I realized I constantly needed them by my side. If I didn't take them, I'd swell up. I couldn't survive without my pills, so I became obsessed with them. When I traveled, I wouldn't check my luggage because I was afraid the airline would lose my pills.

That's when I started to look for other solutions. I tried everything. I visited witch doctors. I took mud baths. I tried acupuncture. You name it, I tried it. The only thing I didn't do was to examine what I put in my mouth. Deep down I knew that what I was eating probably had something to do with my illness. But there's a difference between knowing and doing. Before I knew it, I was 310 pounds. I was still taking high doses of steroids, day and night. I was a cheeseburger away from a heart attack, and I said, "No more. You've got to do something about this, Joe. You're not as smart as you thought you were."

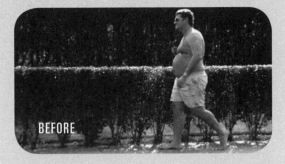

BEFORE

I guess the way I look at it was that I had turned my back on Mother Nature, and I wanted to conduct an experiment where I was the lab rat. What would happen if I ran toward her? Would she open her arms and embrace me, and would I be healed?

I went straight to juicing and a plant-based diet, and within ten to fifteen days the fog started to lift and I was on the path to health. Over the next sixty days, I lost close to 80 pounds and I took my steroid dosage down to zero. That was three and a half years ago, and I haven't touched those pills since.

❯ Joe Cross is the director of *Fat, Sick, and Nearly Dead*, his documentary about regaining his health, and the founder of Reboot Your Life, a socially conscious health and wellness company that helps people change their eating habits. His website is jointhereboot.com.

Water: Liquid Life

No conversation about food is complete without water. A simple glass of water is an essential part of your daily diet. A glass of water travels down your esophagus into your stomach, then through your small intestine, where it's immediately absorbed into your bloodstream. Think about that. Within an hour, the water you just drank will be in your blood.

Water is essential for absorbing nutrients, eliminating waste, and carrying out all cellular activity and actions necessary for life. Without it, you get dehydrated and your body is unable to expel toxins, which causes a tremendous amount of stress on your system. Alcohol, caffeine, soda, and fruit juices high in sugar rob your body of its natural water reserves, leading to adverse effects on your physical, emotional, and mental well-being. According to Daniel Vitalis, "Common ailments and illnesses that are often the result of long-term chronic dehydration include heart disease, fatigue, high blood pressure, headaches, diabetes, and obesity."

Water really is a tremendous source of life.

Once upon a time, water was considered sacred, an almost spiritual element. People used to drink and conserve water with a reverence worthy of a primal source of life. Today, in contrast, we hardly think about water at all. Not only do we drink less and less water, it seems the only time we even notice water is when it's too cold during our morning shower or while we're washing dishes.

"We're at this place in history when people don't believe water matters," according to Daniel Vitalis. "We've kind of desecrated the most sacred thing on the planet. This is crazy, because water is literally what we're made of. The water we drink is a part of our bodies. It's part of our blood. Water matters. It's not just an inert chemical."

Because water is such an important component of our health and well-being, we need to make sure the water we're putting into our systems is clean and fresh. Otherwise our cells are swimming in a toxic soup.

Vitalis believes that it is kind of like a fish tank. "What's more important: the quality of the food you give the fish or the quality of the water in their tank? It's the quality of the water. You wouldn't put dirty water in a fish tank and then go out and buy the highest-quality fish flakes on the market for them, because unless the water's clean, the best food in the world's not going to help them.

"If fish live in polluted water, their systems are polluted. To get the pollutant out of the fish, you have to replace the water. Well, it's the same thing for humans."

The human body is more than 60 percent water. Our blood, our intracellular fluid, our extracellular fluid, and every other kind of fluid in our bodies are made up of the water we drink.

"If you're not drinking extremely clean water," says Vitalis, "then your body's going to take in and bio-accumulate the toxins found in the bad water. Things like the plastics in bottled water. Or fluoride and chlorine, which are added to industrial water and tap water. Or phosphoric acid and lye, which are added to sources of water to balance out the pH levels. All of these things and more get into your cells.

"Switching to a clean water source or high-quality, filtered water lets your cells start to flush out toxins."

Believe it or not, there's a great deal of debate about the best kind of water to drink. Some people don't have access to clean sources of water, generally found in underground aquifers and natural springs. "We've contaminated so many of our natural water sources, it's now really hard to find clean water anywhere on earth," Vitalis says. "Only people with artesian wells or people with direct access to a spring can get to clean water. If neither of those options is realistic, probably the best alternative is to purchase a really good filter or high-quality bottled waters."

Even without the optimal source of fresh water at your fingertips, it's important to remember that your body needs water. Without it, your body will literally die of thirst. Though you might not necessarily feel thirsty, you still need to drink plenty of water.

Kicking Caffeine

Instead of water, most people today reach for coffee, soda, and alcohol. While these beverages do contain water, they are actually diuretics, which means they purge water from the body. When you consume these drinks, your body requires more water than usual to make up for this loss. To ensure that your body continues to function at a high level, replace coffee and soda with natural alternatives that won't draw hydration out of your body.

While small amounts of coffee won't kill you, caffeine can be very addictive and, when consumed in large quantities, can lead to adrenal fatigue. If you want the coffee taste without the addiction, try roasted dandelion root or chicory tea. Herbal or fresh lemon and ginger teas are also great alternatives to coffee. Plus, they can also aid in weight loss and help increase immunity.

If you're not yet ready to give up your morning cup of coffee, make sure you stay properly hydrated, and use organic beans and organic milk whenever possible. Also, replace artificial sweeteners and white sugar with more natural alternatives such as stevia, a natural herb, which actually has a longer-lasting taste than sugar.

"There are now diet drinks with stevia," says Christiane Northrup, M.D., "which is very nice. There's zero sugar and that works. I'm really kind of happy the way the industry has moved forward to give us alternatives that are healthy."

For a quick thirst quencher, squeeze half a lemon into a glass of water, add a pinch of unrefined sea salt, and grate in a half-inch knob of ginger root. Just like that you have a refreshing and healthy glass of lemonade, which will help keep you cool on hot days while also adding nutrients to your body and aiding in detoxification.

If you miss the fizz from soda, add a tablespoon of raw apple cider vinegar—a powerful probiotic—and a squeeze of lemon to sparkling mineral water. It's great for dinner parties.

Healthy Beverage Comparison Chart

LESS HEALTHY

Diet sodas

Sodas

Flavored sports drinks

Vitamin drinks

Bottled pasteurized fruit juices

Coffee

Tap water (often contains fluoride and other contaminates)

Naturally fermented kombucha tea

Freshly squeezed vegetable and fruit juices

Herbal teas

Filtered water

MORE HEALTHY Spring water from source

The Skinny on Milk

According to the old saying, milk does a body good. While this can be true, it really depends on the kind of milk you're drinking and your ability to digest it. And we're not talking about skim, 1 percent, 2 percent, or whole milk. Most of the milk found in your local supermarket is the by-product of modern—and less-than-healthy—feeding and breeding practices of the dairy industry. Rather than letting cows graze naturally on pastures, many dairy farmers confine their stock to concrete stalls and feed them a diet of genetically modified non-organic soy, corn, wheat, hay, and molasses—foods that cows do not naturally digest well. On top of this many farmers also inject cows with growth hormones to help expedite the growing process and increase milk production. Many cows become sick, often due to their unnatural diet and enclosed confines, and are then administered antibiotics to keep them healthy enough to produce milk regularly. Inevitably traces of these hormones and antibiotics end up in our milk.

Then we pasteurize it. Pasteurization can kill harmful bacteria and pathogens present in commercially produced milk. However, it also destroys many nutrients and naturally valuable enzymes like lactase and galactase, which help the human body better digest the lactose and calcium.

According to David Wolfe in *Eating for Beauty,* "Dairy products, based on their high alkaline mineral content, are a health product 'IF' you can digest them. This is a capital 'IF,' as not many of us have the enzymes and gut bacteria necessary to digest them. Pasteurized cow milk and cheeses are mucus forming, as pasteurization destroys the beneficial probiotic cultures that naturally help us to break down the milk and extract the minerals.

"Yogurt is pasteurized and then cultured, so it does contain some probiotic cultures, making it easier to digest. Kefir is generally not pasteurized and therefore contains the largest amount of beneficial probiotic cultures of any dairy product," says Wolfe. "Unpasteurized goat milk, goat cheese, and goat kefir are even easier to digest, contain a higher quantity of alkaline minerals, and are closer to human milk in their composition."

Healthy Milk Comparison Chart

LESS HEALTHY Conventional ultra heat-treated (UHT) milk or milk powder

Conventional pasteurized and homogenized milk

Organic pasteurized and homogenized milk

Organic pasture-raised cow or goat milk

MORE HEALTHY Organic cow or goat milk kefir (cultured milk)

Note: Healthy dairy-free milk alternatives include Homemade Coconut Milk (page 125) and Nut Milk (page 126) and hemp-seed, oat, and rice milks.

CHAPTER FIVE

You Are What You Think

Emotional Eating and Childhood Cravings

In 1992, Vincent Felitti, M.D., head of the Department of Preventive Medicine at Kaiser Permanente in San Diego, noticed a number of his patients dropping out of Kaiser's obesity program. The patients, Felitti noticed, didn't quit because they couldn't lose weight. What was going on? Why were his patients dropping out? To answer these questions, Felitti conducted a research project. Through his study—popularly known as the Adverse Childhood Experiences (ACE) study—Felitti discovered that a high proportion of the dropouts had histories of childhood abuse or neglect. These childhood experiences, he concluded, continued to affect his patients' health and well-being, even if the experiences had occurred more than fifty years earlier.

"What he concluded," says Christiane Northrup, M.D., "is that obesity is not the problem. It's a solution. It's a solution to chronic stress. It's a solution in many people to sexual abuse, to dysfunctional family situations, and other personal traumas."

Overeating is often an indication that we're coping with some known—or unknown—problem or stress. And when we overeat, we go right for the kinds of foods we ate as children, foods packed with sugar and empty calories, but which resonate with us for one reason or another. The emotional eating habits we pick up as adults are rooted in intense cravings left over from our childhoods.

"It's not just what you're eating," says Kris Carr. "It's also what's eating you. When people are stressed or sad, they often turn to food for comfort, especially foods that they ate growing up: meat loaf, mashed potatoes, cake, cookies—all those things that you ate or your mom made for you. The foods that may remind us of a time when we were nurtured and nourished."

This kind of emotional eating is extremely common, according to Jon Gabriel. "I've talked to so many people who have been overweight all their lives and I always ask them, 'When did it start?' They usually respond, 'When I was four years old.' Well, what happened when they were four years old? 'My father was an alcoholic and he beat me,' or 'We moved to another country and I was really scared.' I heard this all the time."

These kinds of mental and emotional stresses make the body believe it's under attack. And as we've seen, once the body believes it's at risk, it immediately tries to protect itself, because that's what it's designed to do. "Weight gain can be associated with specific types of stress that you wouldn't normally ever associate with weight gain," Gabriel says. "Sleep deprivation, dehydration, mental and emotional stress, fighting traffic, worrying about your job or your boss or how you're going to pay your mortgage or credit card bills—all of these types of stress cause a chemical reaction in your body that's basically the same as the stress caused by a famine. When that chemistry is the same as a famine, your body wants to gain weight to protect you from the stresses in your life. It doesn't know what else to do.

"We get so mad at our bodies, because we think our bodies are trying to sabotage us, that our bodies are out to get us. They're not. The weight gain is a protection mechanism. It's nothing more."

Once we understand that sudden weight gain is often the result of the body's protection mechanism, we can start to deactivate this mechanism by addressing specific stresses in our lives.

"Look at where you're not satisfied," Carr suggests. "Are you in a dead-end job? Are you married to somebody who treats you like dirt? Are you suffocating under the weight of too much pressure in your life? Are there residual traumas and dramas that need to be attended to? Is there some unfinished business that's keeping you stuck and will ultimately encourage you to make poor food choices?

"One of the best pieces of advice I ever got from a spiritual teacher was this: if you're upset, don't eat. And I think it's so profound because oftentimes when we're upset we have no connection to whether or not we're satiated or whether or not we're full. Because we're trying to fill a void that can never be filled with food."

Stress and Stress Reduction

When you're under stress, your body produces stress hormones called cortisol and epinephrine. The presence of cortisol and epinephrine, particularly in excessive amounts, can prevent your body from processing fat. "If you've ever seen someone on steroid medications, such as prednisone, you see that the first thing that happens is they gain 20 or 30 pounds, no matter what they're eating," says Dr. Northrup. "In fact, when your stress cortisol hormone levels are high enough, they've documented that looking at a doughnut actually changes your metabolism."

> *"When your stress cortisol hormone levels are high enough,*
> *they've documented that looking at a doughnut*
> *actually changes your metabolism."*
>
> —DR. CHRISTIANE NORTHRUP

"Stress also increases fluid retention," Dr. Northrup continues. "I call those liquid pounds. If you're under stress and you sleep for only three to four hours a night, you will gain two pounds just from that. You want to take care of those liquid pounds before they turn into real pounds, which they inevitably will."

The easiest and most effective way to digest stress hormones is through deep sleep. A good night's sleep will metabolize, or break down, excess cortisol and epinephrine better than anything else.

Exercise also helps the body break down these stress hormones. A walk three or four times a week is all it takes. "When you lift weights or you simply take a long walk," Dr. Northrup says, "you increase all those feel-good hormones you usually turn to sugar for, and this is as good as antidepressants for mild to moderate depression. I mean this is insane. You just exercise alone and know that when you get out there and you're in the fresh air, you feel much better."

THREE EASY STEPS TO REDUCE STRESS

1. **Sleep deeply**

   Get to bed early, darken your room, turn off nearby electrical equipment, and reduce any excess noises.

2. **Exercise**

   Walk in the fresh air and breathe deeply into your abdomen, making sure to expand your belly. This draws oxygen into your cells and helps to relax the body.

3. **Laugh**

   Watch funny movies, read a book that makes you laugh out loud, spend time with friends who make you giggle—anything that puts you in a good mood.

"Anything that is sustainably pleasurable will decrease stress hormones," Dr. Northrup continues. "Laughter decreases them enormously, and that's been clinically shown to improve immunity and also decrease pain. I recommend you have some funny movies lying around."

Visualization

It's almost impossible to lose weight or change your body if you can't even start to imagine the type of body you want. This is sometimes hard for people to understand, but think about it: Can you redesign your living room or bedroom if you don't know what kind of furniture you want or what color you want to paint the walls? The first step is imagining the room. The second step is bringing that vision to life.

Well, the same is true for dieting and weight loss. Visualization is a vital part of the process.

"A lot of people look at my before and after pictures," says Jon Gabriel, author of *The Gabriel Method*, "and they wonder how I lost all this weight without any type of surgery. I can tell you, the body I have now is exactly the body I visualized having when I was 200 pounds overweight. That's not a coincidence."

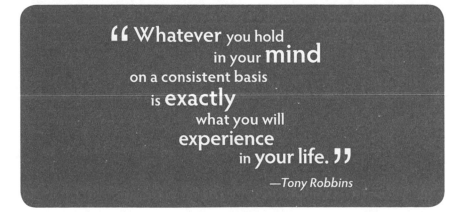

❝ Whatever you hold
in your **mind**
on a consistent basis
is **exactly**
what you will
experience
in **your life. ❞**

—*Tony Robbins*

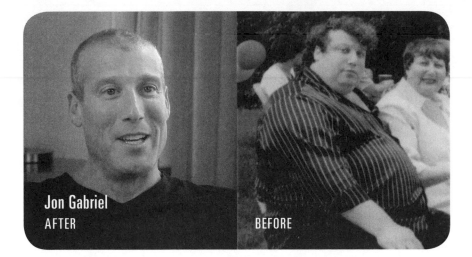

Jon Gabriel
AFTER
BEFORE

Visualization, according to Gabriel, is like a language you can use to talk to your subconscious, or the unconscious part of your brain that lets your body know that it's time to lose weight. "You can't talk to someone who doesn't speak your language. Say you have to go to the bathroom in a foreign country. You could ask a thousand people where the bathroom is, but they won't tell you because they don't know what you're asking them. But if you draw a picture of a bathroom on a napkin, they instantly know what you mean. Visualization, or symbols, in this case is the universal language for people who don't speak your language. Well, your body doesn't speak your language. But it can recognize an image."

To help your body understand your body goals, Gabriel suggests finding a picture of a body you'd like to have. The picture can be of yourself when you were in better shape or it could be somebody else. It doesn't matter. You just have to look at it. "Just look at the picture for thirty seconds in a subconscious way," he says. "Don't look at it with your eyes. Look through it to let your subconscious absorb it for thirty seconds or so. Then close your eyes and see yourself, feel yourself, and imagine yourself being in that body, imagine yourself walking on the beach with that body—whatever way you can do it."

Eventually, your subconscious will start to understand what you want. It will start to figure out how to calm the internal stresses that lead to weight gain. "Your subconscious will begin to understand that it doesn't need all this fat," Gabriel says. "It will understand that it doesn't have to hold on to all this fat because of some imagined famine or trauma. It will slowly realize it's been confusing these stresses, because it never really understood what to do with the stresses in modern-day life. 'Do I get fatter? Do I get thinner? How do I protect this scared person?' Normally, it would preserve fat. But when you communicate with your subconscious, you can tell it that's not what you need, and it will turn off the fat programs. And that's when everything starts to change."

While visualization can help in weight loss, it basically acts like a muscle. It will only get stronger if you use it. Make visualization a regular habit. While going about your day, picture yourself with the body you want. "When you're walking to work or sitting at your desk, just imagine your body is in perfect shape. Your subconscious will respond."

The two best times to practice visualization are first thing in the morning and right before bed. This is when your mind is in its most relaxed state and you are easily able to access your subconscious.

To download a free evening visualization audio MP3 with Jon Gabriel, visit www.HungryForChange.tv/bonuses.

The Four-Letter Word

Unfortunately, most of us start our days on the wrong foot. As soon as we get out of the shower, we look in the mirror and only see all of our minor and not-so-minor imperfections. Our skin is blotchy. Our arms are flabby. Our stomachs stick out too far or sag. So what happens? We

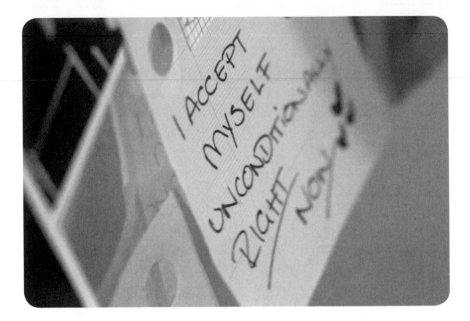

spend the rest of the day berating ourselves for everything we think is wrong. "How could I let it get this bad?" we think. "How could anyone ever find me attractive?" we ask. "I'm not worthy of love or affection," we tell ourselves.

Would we put up with a person whispering these things into our ears every day? Of course not. And yet we do it to ourselves constantly, sometimes as often as every minute of every day. "I don't know about you, but that type of person wouldn't last five minutes with me," says Joe Cross, director of the film *Fat, Sick, and Nearly Dead*. "Yet we allow ourselves to do it to ourselves."

Such thoughts, according to Dr. Christiane Northrup, prevent us from getting what we want or feeling the way we want—and deserve—to feel. "I actually think that the concept of loving yourself is key to all of it," she says. "Without that, nothing else is going to be sustainable.

"Louise Hay of Hay House has a really wonderful practice, and I have been prescribing it to my patients for years. I tell them to write this message on a piece of paper and tape it to their mirrors and repeat

> *"If we had a rampant epidemic of self-love,*
> *then our healthcare costs would go down dramatically."*
> —DR. CHRISTIANE NORTHRUP

it twice a day, in the morning and again at night. The message is simple. 'I accept myself unconditionally right now.' If you do this for thirty days, by about day twenty-eight something shifts inside and you begin to believe these words, because you are planting a new affirmation."

Just as you need to practice visualization regularly for it to work, so too do you need to say out loud personal affirmations as often as possible, so these thoughts start to take root. The more you hear these words of encouragement and self-worth, the more you will believe them. The more you believe them, the healthier you'll get.

"As a doctor, let me tell you what self-love does," says Dr. Northrup. "It improves your hearing and your eyesight. It lowers your blood pressure. It increases pulmonary function and cardiac output. It helps wire in the musculature. If we had a rampant epidemic of self-love, then our healthcare costs would go down dramatically. This isn't just some froufrou New Age notion. This is hardcore science."

> **" I am** by nature
> a dealer in **words,**
> and words are the most
> **powerful drug**
> known to **humanity. "**
>
> —*Rudyard Kipling, 1865–1936*

Profile in Health

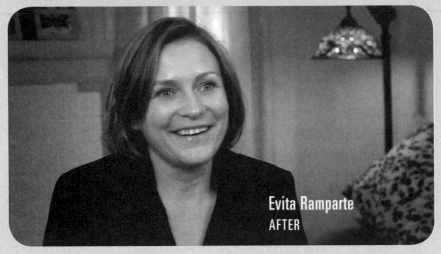

Evita Ramparte
AFTER

I grew up in Poland. My family and I ate a lot of sausages and pierogi, traditional Polish food, which is all very oily. After Communism collapsed in Poland, we started eating American food, like pizza, fast food, and potato chips. We had no idea about our health or how to eat. No one ever told us fast food is bad for you. When I was a girl, I was overweight. I was shy and chronically depressed. My face was very blotchy. I had a horrible complexion. School was very stressful for me. I felt like I was a circle, a big round thing, and I was being pushed into a square and I had to fit in. And I didn't like it. In gym class, I was always the last person picked. When we had to run or sprint, my class would point and laugh. They said I wasn't running, I was rolling. As a teenager, no one ever noticed me. I could never get the attention of boys because they were swept away by my girlfriends. They never looked twice at me.

Later, when I finally got married, I was still kind of depressed; I had a toxic mind-set. I wasn't fulfilled at all, and my husband and I were not happy. I was a sugar and coffee junkie. I would wake up every morning, open my eyes, then go right for a very strong cup of coffee, because I couldn't wake up. I didn't want to get out of bed. I needed certain foods in order to stay sane, but I always felt like my energy was spiraling down the drain. Life just wasn't fun. I felt like I was wrapped in a blanket with three holes in it—two to watch television and one to eat. In fact, the only fun I had was watching people on TV having fun. It was like I was on a train, and life was passing by outside of the window. I remember thinking, please stop this train. I'm getting off. If this is called life, I want off.

Before things got better, they got worse. I was diagnosed with ovarian cancer, but I used my sickness as an opportunity to make a change. I decided to experiment, because I was fighting for my life. What else did I have to lose? What if it works? So I went to the farmers' market and bought a lot of vegetables: beets and kale and all sorts of things. At first, they didn't look attractive to me, but I stuck with it for three days. All I did was juicing and enemas, detoxing my body of all the sugar, caffeine, and chemicals. After three days, I lost around 15 pounds, and my skin cleared up for the first time in my life. It was also the first time I ever lost weight naturally, and so fast. I tried a whole bunch of other weight-loss programs, but they never worked. But after the cleanse and just three days of juicing, my pants were getting loose and my tongue started to respond to veggies and avocado, and I discovered a whole new set of flavors, natural flavors that I never tasted before. I felt like I was beginning a new life.

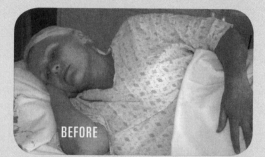

BEFORE

I slowly started to heal myself physically. Within four months, I was cancer-free and I'd lost 83 pounds. My friends didn't recognize me. I was like a butterfly that came out of its cocoon.

After I healed, I discovered my natural beauty. And I discovered my body, and I started to move, and I started to feel a lot of joy in doing sports. When you take care of yourself, something powerful happens. You realize you're precious. You fall in love with yourself, and that love shines through you and overflows to others. You give yourself permission to live how you want to live.

> Evita Ramparte is a leading health journalist, holistic coach, and media producer. She transformed her health through juicing and a plant-based diet after an ovarian cancer diagnosis in 2000. She's been interviewed by MTV Europe and *Cosmopolitan* magazine, and she empowers people to transform their own health. Her website is www.evitaramparte.com.

Profile in Health

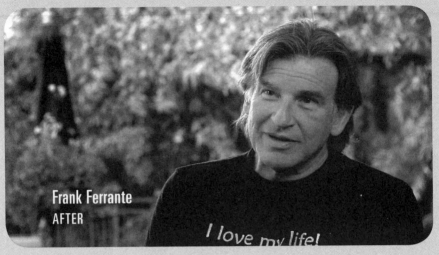

Frank Ferrante
AFTER

I love my life!

I n the 1990s, I was diagnosed with hepatitis C. I had started dating someone, and we decided to get tested for HIV and other sexually transmitted diseases. Initially, the test came back clean, which in all honesty amazed me, because I was a recovering alcoholic and drug addict and precaution wasn't exactly my strong suit back then. Two weeks later, however, the clinic called me back and told me they had made a mistake. I had hepatitis C. This hit me really hard. Instead of turning back to drugs or alcohol, I started using food. It was very incremental. It was like suicide on the installment plan. I was taking my time destroying myself. Of course, I wasn't conscious of it. It wasn't like a shot of vodka, like whenever I felt anxious I consciously thought to have a drink. A food addiction is much more insidious. It sneaks up on you, more so than booze, because everybody's eating and there are just so many people who are overweight and there are so many people who look like you and are doing what you're doing. I started to get depressed and I started to let myself go bit by bit. By the time I realized how much I had let myself go, I was completely overwhelmed.

People who have never been overweight have no idea what it's like to be obese. There are so many aspects of being fat that are dispiriting. Each one affects every aspect of your life, everything from your self-esteem and emotional well-being to your wardrobe to your hygiene. Before I lost the weight, I was over 300 pounds.

When I woke up in the morning, I was immediately aware of my body and I was immediately aware that I didn't like it. When you're that overweight, you don't feel seen or heard. Nobody wants anything to do with you. Believe it or not, I used to ring my own doorbell to hear what it would sound like if a visitor stopped by. Death seemed at least a welcome prospect. I wasn't suicidal, but I occasionally had dark thoughts about death. You know, like "just turn the switch. Turn it off, flip the off button. I'm ready for the Big Sleep, man." My head was filled

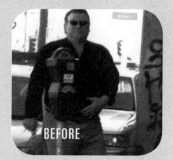
BEFORE

with all those voices that would tell me I was worthless. That I was a slob or a pig. That no one would ever love me. The depth of my self-loathing was bottomless.

But here's the thing. The ultimate act of sanity and responsibility is taking care of yourself.

Eventually, I got turned on to raw food by a group of people who wanted to help me turn my life around. What did I know about raw food? I just imagined carrots and celery with ranch dressing. How could I possibly be vegan? I thought Vegan was a planet. But I kept at it. After about two weeks, I noticed my energy started coming back. Colors appeared brighter. I felt just a little bit lighter in my step.

The biggest change, however, came in how I felt about myself. As I improved my diet, I started to learn to love myself—probably for the first time ever. You probably want to know the most important part to losing and keeping off weight. You probably want to know the crucial component. Well, let me tell you: It is, without question, love. Love for myself and love for other people. It's all about self-love. The group of people who helped me used to tell me, "Let us love you till you love yourself." When I first heard that, I got so sad. I didn't even know how little I cared about myself. Letting someone love me actually hurt. It was physically painful. It was at this point when the genesis of willingness emerges. I was ready to make a change. It was just a crack but, as Leonard Cohen says, the cracks let the light in. That crack, that ability to love myself unconditionally, let the light in.

> Frank Ferrante is the subject of the documentary *May I Be Frank*. A lover of life, great food, beautiful women, and a good laugh, Frank was also a drug addict, morbidly obese, prediabetic, and fighting hepatitis C. *May I Be Frank* documents the transformation of Frank Ferrante's life. His website is mayibefrankferrante.com.

Profile in Health

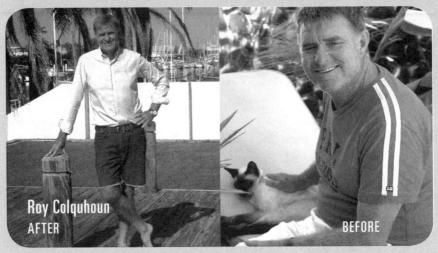

Roy Colquhoun
AFTER

BEFORE

In 2002, my health was in a poor state. I was overweight. I consumed an unhealthy meat- and dairy-based diet, and I drank too much alcohol. It seemed I was constantly suffering from severe flu-like symptoms. To make matters worse, I worked long hours in my own business as a chartered accountant and registered company auditor. I was totally unaware that I was in a highly stressed, constant fight-or-flight state for what turned out to be a period of many years. This heightened level of stress and anxiety had become my normal state. I had become so conditioned to my on-edge state I couldn't even remember what it felt like to feel good.

During the summer of 2003, I suffered from total adrenal exhaustion. My body literally shut down. For months on end I was bedridden and too ill to get up. I thought I had contracted a rare tropical disease. At the time, my medical practitioner diagnosed me with chronic fatigue syndrome. He prescribed for me antidepressants and referred me to a psychiatrist. I didn't think twice about his diagnosis. I mean, why should I have? Where else was I going to turn? Because of my professional background, I was convinced the answer to my ongoing health problems would come from the mainstream medical profession. In my determination to get myself well again, I sought out a whole range of specialists and traditional medical practitioners, including psychiatrists and psychologists. They put me on a cocktail of antidepressants, antipsychotics, anxiety medication, and sleeping tablets. My life was a psychotic daze. I was spiraling out of control. My psychiatrist admitted me to a psychiatric hospital for thirty days of evaluation. Even this didn't help. I was released with a new cocktail of prescription medications.

Eventually, I had to sell my business and retire from the workforce. I felt helpless and hopelessness. Nothing the medical profession prescribed worked. I didn't think I had anywhere else to turn. Suicide was becoming a frightening and very real option.

This was until my son and daughter-in-law James and Laurentine showed up on my doorstep with a rough copy of their new documentary, FOOD MATTERS. They told me they weren't leaving until I recovered. Stay as long as you want, I remember thinking when they showed up. I'm not going to get any better. The best medical professionals in Australia could not help me. How could my son and daughter-in-law with their nutrition- and vitamin-based diet? With some not-so-gentle persuasion from my loving wife, Megan, I hesitantly decided to give James and Laurentine a chance. They immediately recommended a clinical dose of vitamins to replace all my prescription medications. And they put me on a ten-day cleanse, during which time I ate only raw, plant-based foods and stopped drinking alcohol.

After five years of antidepressants, antipsychotics, anxiety medication, and sleeping tablets, I decided to quit them cold turkey, replacing them with clinical doses of vitamins. My medical specialists had all warned me against going off my medications, telling me I would experience major withdrawal symptoms. Maybe I was just lucky or maybe I had the right clinical amount of vitamins, because I am still waiting for the withdrawal symptoms to kick in five years later.

The statement on the cover of the HUNGRY FOR CHANGE DVD is "Your Health Is in Your Hands." This isn't just a marketing slogan. It's a profound endorsement of the amazing ability to heal yourself naturally, without the aid of drugs or surgery. If I had not replaced all the prescription medications with a plant-based diet, natural supplements, and other lifestyle changes, I honestly don't believe I would be alive today. But here I am at age fifty-seven, 55 pounds lighter than I was at the depths of my despair and ill health. I am the fittest I have ever been, running twenty-five to thirty miles a week. I am now fully recovered and loving life again.

CHAPTER SIX

Eating for Beauty

The History of Attraction

Everybody wants to look good. And let's face it. Nothing looks better than being healthy and fit. As a species, we're programmed to be attracted to the people who look good. Why? Because the best-looking ones are usually the healthiest ones. "We are naturally designed to screen each other for health for reproductive purposes," says Daniel Vitalis, leading traditional- and wild-foods expert. "We look at each other and we see glowing skin, we see shining eyes, and that's sexy to us. A confident person is sexy to us."

The skin is a true symbol of health, because it's an outward reflection of what's going on right beneath the surface. Nutrients push their way from the inside of the body out through the skin, which gives a person a recognizable glow, which lets others know on an instinctual level that a person probably has a healthy liver, kidneys, lungs, and heart.

"People look for symmetry," says David Wolfe, a leading nutrition expert and author of *Eating for Beauty*. "They look for a steady skin tone

THE SUNSHINE VITAMIN

When we expose our skin to sunlight, our bodies respond in kind. The sun's UVB rays produce within us vitamin D, a natural vitamin and hormone. As a natural product of sunlight, vitamin D supercharges the cells in our bodies.

The major biological function of vitamin D, according to Mike Adams, is to maintain normal blood levels of calcium and phosphorus. "Vitamin D helps us absorb calcium, and thus helps to form and maintain strong bones and teeth," he says. "Without vitamin D, bones start to become thin, brittle, soft, or misshapen."

By limiting our time in the sun, due to its perceived danger, we deprive our bodies of many essential vitamins and nutrients required for optimal health.

"Vitamin D is also essential for losing weight," says Jon Gabriel, author of *The Gabriel Method*. "Vitamin D turns off our bodies' fat programs, and a lack of vitamin D turns on the fat programs. In winter, when there's not enough sun, the body thinks there isn't enough food, so it turns on its fat programs.

"The sun is our life force. It is our connection to life itself."

There are numerous studies that have demonstrated the connection between full-spectrum light and serotonin, a neurotransmitter widely believed to be a major contributor to happiness, energy, and general well-being.

"Interestingly, a drop in melatonin enhances feel-good hormones, including endorphins and serotonin, which help you feel both alert and calm," says Dr. Christiane Northrup. "This transformation occurs in the brain as a result of being in more light. That's why getting outside at noon for a half-hour walk on a sunny day during the winter months will lift your mood greatly.

"So let the sun in whenever you can, especially during the winter. Safe exposure to the sun, coupled with a regular dose of vitamin D (2,000 to 5,000 IU per day) will do wonders for your health all year long."

and not a lot of splotchy type of colors on your skin. That's what we're all striving for: a deep richness of skin tone, a deep richness of hair, a luster in our nails, an overall feeling of shine and glow. Why? Well, it makes us look younger and sexier, and those are the cues that we pick up on as humans. This is built into our definition of beauty, and this is why the beauty industry spends so much time and money trying to create products that help our skin look artificially monotone."

Unfortunately, most skin creams and other beauty products often contain toxins and chemicals designed to give people an instant "natural looking" glow.

"There are all different types of synthetic compounds that make it into the cosmetic industry," according to Wolfe, "like sodium lauryl sulfate and other sudsing agents that are used in detergents, shampoos, and body lotions. We're talking about lead compounds, mercury compounds, and even compounds like urea, which is made from horse urine."

"The typical over-the-counter skin cream contains dozens of potentially harmful toxins," says Mike Adams, a consumer health advocate and editor of NaturalNews.com, who recently analyzed a popular perfume product. "It contained twenty-one different potentially carcinogenic chemicals, none of which are listed on the label. So you have to ask yourself, do you want your skin to be treated with nutrition from the inside out? Or do you want to coat your skin with petrochemicals and toxic chemicals and artificial fragrance products from the outside, which your body will absorb into your liver and your heart and your kidneys and your brain?

"Which way would you rather deal with your skin? Which way is going to make you look better in the long run? Which way are you going to be sexier?"

"Sometimes people have skin issues," says David Wolfe. "They'll have blemishes on their face, eczema, acne, psoriasis, or any number of other difficulties. These blotches or irritations are external signs that your body

TWELVE HARMFUL COSMETIC INGREDIENTS

1. Sodium laureth sulphate and sodium lauryl sulphate

Used in some foaming cosmetics, such as shampoos, cleansers, and bubble bath, sodium laureth sulphate can be contaminated with 1,4-dioxane, which may cause cancer.

2. Paraben, methylparaben, butylparaben, and propylparaben

Used in a variety of cosmetics as preservatives, these chemicals are suspected endocrine disrupters and may interfere with male reproductive functions.

3. Petrolatum

Used in some hair products for shine and as a moisture barrier in some lip balms, lipsticks, and moisturizers, petrolatum and other petroleum-based products can be contaminated with polycyclic aromatic hydrocarbons, which may cause cancer.

4. Coal-tar dyes

Coal-tar dyes include p-phenylenediamine (PPD) and colors listed as "CI" (color index) followed by five numbers (such as CI 15510). They are used in hair and other dyes and may be contaminated with heavy metals toxic to the brain.

5. Butylated hydroxyanisole (BHA) and butylated hydroxytoluene (BHT)

Used in moisturizers as preservatives, BHA and BHT, as suspected endocrine disrupters, may cause cancer. They are known to be harmful to fish and other wildlife.

6. Diethanolamine (DEA), cocamide DEA, and lauramide DEA

Used in some creamy and foaming moisturizers and shampoos, these amides react to nitrosamines, which may cause cancer. They are harmful to fish and other wildlife.

7. Dibutyl phthalate

Used as a plasticizer in some nail-care products, dibutyl phthalate, is a suspected endocrine disrupter and a reproductive toxicant. It is harmful to fish and other wildlife.

8. DMDM hydantoin, diazolidinyl urea, imidazolidinyl urea, methenamine, quaternium-15, and sodium hydroxymethylglycinate

Used in a variety of cosmetics, these preservatives slowly release small amounts of formaldehyde, which causes cancer.

9. Perfume

Some fragrances, like perfume, can trigger allergies and asthma. Some are even linked to cancer and neurotoxicity and are harmful to fish and other wildlife.

10. PEG compounds

Used in some cosmetic cream bases, PEG compounds (such as PEG-60) can be contaminated with 1,4-dioxane, which may cause cancer.

11. Siloxanes: cyclotetrasiloxane, cyclopentasiloxane, cyclohexasiloxane, and cyclomethicone

Used in a variety of cosmetics to soften, smooth, and moisten, siloxanes are suspected endocrine disrupters and, in the case of cyclotetrasiloxane, a reproductive toxicant. They are harmful to fish and other wildlife.

12. Triclosan

Used in some antibacterial cosmetics, such as toothpastes, cleansers, and deodorants, triclosan is a suspected endocrine disrupter and may contribute to antibiotic resistance in bacteria. It is harmful to fish and other wildlife.

Information courtesy of the David Suzuki Foundation, www.cbc.ca/news/story/2010/10/19/suzuki-dirty-dozen.html.

is inflamed and may be trying to rid itself of toxins in any way it can." What many people may not realize is the skin is the largest organ in the body and one of the primary ways that the body eliminates toxins.

"We're constantly being barraged with the idea that technology is the way to sexy," says Daniel Vitalis. "Whether that's medical intervention or whether that's pharmaceutically based or whether that's some kind of pharmaceutically enhanced longevity cream we put on our faces. But really these things come from nature. Caring for our skin is pretty simple.

"The skin lives on oils, like coconut oil and olive oil, and other food-grade oils. We see this all over the world. We see it in ancient Rome and Greece, where they applied olive oil to their skin. We see this in Polynesia today, where they cover their bodies in coconut oil. It's not hard to look and be sexy."

Beauty is the product of a good diet. Different foods affect us differently, and what we put in our mouths, what we can digest and eliminate, and how our bodies handle toxins all affect our appearance.

"Let's take vanity," says Dr. Northrup, "because it's a very good entryway to healthy living. Your skin looks better when you are eating a diet that is low-glycemic, where the blood sugar is stable. Your skin, your hair, your nails begin to look better. One of the reasons that I personally stopped eating so many grains and high-glycemic foods over the years was that I noticed a couple things. First of all, I noticed weight gain, every year a little more and every year harder and harder to keep off. Second of all, my patients and I all started to have fingernails that broke, hair that broke, and skin that was getting all red. When you eat well, those problems start to go away."

What most people don't realize is that the same diet that prevents diabetes and heart disease also leads to a radiant complexion. A diet too high in refined carbohydrates, for example, or highly oxidized foods like fried or barbecued foods, ages us from the inside out.

If you want your skin to appear more youthful, according to Dr. Northrup, you'll need plenty of vitamin C, a powerful anti-oxidant and anti-aging vitamin, and essential fatty acids.

"Essential fatty acids are found in nuts and seeds, whole grains, eggs, and good-quality fish and poultry—foods that are healthy for the entire body as well as the skin," she says. "The typical American diet is deficient in healthy omega-3 fats. And fish oil, a terrific source of omega-3 fatty acids, is one of the best beauty supplements for skin, hair, and nails."

Healthy vegetarian sources of omega-3 essential fatty acids include chia seeds, flaxseeds, and various types of algae.

The truth is, you really can eat yourself sexy. Because physical beauty is an outward manifestation of inner cleanliness, proper nutrition leads to the healthy, vibrant look everyone so desperately wants. If you eat the right fats and live foods, your skin will undoubtedly start to clear up.

In his book *Eating for Beauty*, David Wolfe describes how certain foods contain specific beautifying qualities. Known as beauty foods, they are filled with high levels of anti-oxidants and anti-inflammatory properties. "A proper diet can make us feel incredible, lead to limitless beauty, and increase longevity," says Wolfe. "Raw plant foods, containing a spectrum of essential vitamins and minerals, can restore elasticity to the tissues. Green leafy vegetables provide fiber and alkalinity to help keep us clean on the inside. Foods high in silicon, iron, and magnesium can restore the mineral density to bones, hair, and teeth and give you glowing skin. Sulfur helps your connective tissue and reverses age-related lines and fills out your protein makeup so that your musculature and your overall build reflect the higher qualities that beauty points to. To eat for beauty, make sure to eat foods like aloe vera, arugula, macadamia nuts, olive oil and olives, cucumbers, and radishes."

Eating lots of fruits, vegetables, and other fresh food, coupled with special beauty foods and natural supplements, will improve your appearance, vitality, and health.

DAVID WOLFE'S TOP BEAUTY MINERALS

Beauty foods contain high concentrations of sulfur, silicon, zinc, iron, and/or manganese.

Sulfur, though often overlooked, is in every cell of the human body, most notably in the joints, hair, skin, and nails. It helps with complexion, healthy hair, glowing skin, and tissue elasticity and maintenance. Foods rich in sulfur include arugula, cabbage, kale, broccoli, mustard leaves, Brussels sprouts, garlic, and horseradish, among others.

Silicon-rich foods help increase bone-mineral density and can prevent cavities, bleeding gums, and gum atrophy. These include alfalfa, romaine lettuce, spinach, burdock root, radishes, cucumber, bell peppers, tomatoes, and oats, among others.

Zinc aids in skin beauty, cell and body growth, sexual development, fertility, vision, taste, and smell. The best sources of zinc include poppy and pumpkin seeds, sunflower seeds, pecans, cashews, macadamia nuts, coconut, spinach, spirulina, and seaweed.

Iron, coupled with hemoglobin, carries oxygen through the body's respiration system. Iron deficiencies lead to light-headedness and fatigue. Some vegetarian iron-rich foods include onions, shallots, cherries, blackberries, collards, parsley, spinach, and most dark green leafy vegetables and red-colored berries.

Manganese helps form cartilage, bone, and connective tissue. It also regulates iron in the blood, helping to improve the oxygenation of the blood, nerves, and brain cells, as required. Some powerful sources of manganese are cloves, cacao beans (raw chocolate), hemp seeds, Brazil nuts, almonds, pecans, spinach, watercress, kale, wild lettuces, raisins, prunes, and sweet potatoes, among others.

Another great way to get beautiful skin is through juicing.

"Fresh juice from vegetables and fruits, which you can make in your own kitchen, will completely turn your skin around in thirty days," says Mike Adams, editor of NaturalNews.com. "Your friends will ask you what's your secret, and when you tell them you've been juicing fresh produce, they'll probably say, 'Well I'm just going to buy a skin cream,' because they want the easier way. But you'll know your juice beats their skin cream.

"That's why people who are going to a class reunion or a family picnic or a wedding, who want to look great and sexy and young and vibrant, . . . are learning the secret to juicing a month or two before the event. By the time it comes around, they look fantastic—and everybody knows it."

Profile in Health

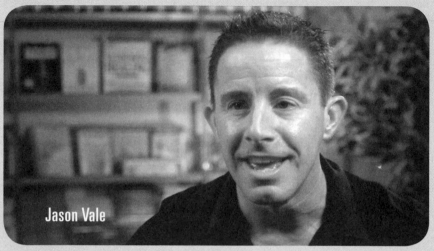

Jason Vale

The thing that made me get into juicing above anything else was my own health. Most people in the diet and juicing industries didn't get here by accident. They're here because they were once ill or had a chronic condition. I used to be covered from head to foot in psoriasis and eczema. I had a hard time finding clear patches of skin. Rashes and blotches covered my neck and my face. They covered the back of my knees. It was so bad I couldn't even wear a pair of jeans. If I did, my skin would crack. Even worse, when I went to sleep, the cracked areas behind my knees would heal overnight, but would then re-crack and ooze pus as soon as I straightened my legs in the morning. It was terrible. On top of all that, I also had really bad asthma and hay fever, so bad I really couldn't go outside whenever it acted up. I needed to lock myself in an airtight room.

Now, I didn't really help matters. I was a heavy drinker and smoker, lighting up forty to sixty cigarettes a day. What can I say? I grew up in Britain. Roll with the punches, right? I also ate anything, at any time, as long as it wasn't green. If it looked healthy, I wouldn't touch it. Instead, I loaded up with fat, salt, and sugar to the point where I was addicted to these things. I was addicted to alcohol, cigarettes, and processed foods. I knew I was physically hurting myself with these things, but I just couldn't stop. Addiction is an invisible prison, and I couldn't break out.

This led me to try to do something about my condition. I was always a science kind of guy, so I started studying how the body worked. I realized my digestive system was all beat up after years of trying to break down all these toxins and chemicals, extract nutrients, and dispose of all the waste from the wrong kinds of food. It turns out this puts a tremendous strain on the digestive system. In the absence of genuine vitamins, minerals, and macro- and micronutrients, the body tries to turn all this bad food into usable food. What happens is you feel bloated and hungry at the same time. You're overfed and undernourished. This is exactly what I was going through. I kept asking myself, How can I still be hungry when I can't even think about eating more food?

So I figured if I couldn't eat it, I'd drink it. This allowed me to "feed" my body on a cellular level through water-rich, organic nutrients and minerals. After drinking a couple of juices a day, I noticed I was hungry less and less. My body was finally getting what it needed. Freshly extracted juice was my fifteen-minute nutrient express to health. It really is the ultimate fast food, because the juice enters your stomach and, within fifteen minutes, all these nutrients and minerals have found their way into your cells. I'm talking about zinc, selenium, the right kind of essential fatty acids, like omega-3, -6, and -9, and things like lecithin granules. Juicing also helps keep you hydrated, which prevents cracked or dry skin.

The level of improvement people see after they start juicing is amazing. Their stomach problems, from irritable bowel syndrome to Crohn's disease, lessen. Their skin clears. Their breathing starts to improve. The body really responds to it. Once you remove refined sugars, refined fats, and junk foods from your diet, once you take out all the wheat, the breads, and the manufactured foods, and replace them with water-rich, organic nutrients and minerals, the body will want more and more and more of it. Your body will tell you, "If you're good to me, I'll be good to you." Your skin will start to glow. Your eyes will start to brighten. Your hair will become thicker and look more vibrant. Your entire body will shine for you.

> Jason Vale is a leading authority on health, addiction, and juicing. His books—*7lbs in 7 Days: Super Juice Diet*, *Juice Master: Turbo-Charge Your Life in 14 Days*, and *Slim for Life*—have sold more than 2 million copies around the world. Jason turned to juicing to transform his own health and is now known as the Juice Master. He helps transform people's health the world over through his books, DVDs, and juice retreats. His website is www.thejuicemaster.com.

We all want more energy. We all want an ideal body. We all want beautiful, younger-looking skin. You can get all of these things by making subtle adjustments to your diet and lifestyle. Just remember, the better you feel about yourself, the better you'll look, and the better you look, the better you'll feel about yourself.

"A lot of people look at me and think that I must be in my twenties," says Kris Carr, author of *Crazy Sexy Diet*. "Well, I'm not, but that's always a nice compliment. I love hearing that people think that I'm a lot younger than I am. I'm heading into my forties and certainly believe that this lifestyle has helped me not only live a healthy life with a chronic disease but also feel younger and more vibrant and—depending on the lighting—look pretty good too."

Ultimately, the pursuit of health and beauty is holistic. Health and beauty are the result of a series of actions and decisions you make over an extended period of time, which take you toward longevity and healthy living. The goal of eating for beauty, really, is about finding a sustainable level of happiness and self-confidence.

"Before I was sick," says Carr, "I thought I had nothing without my health. Then I got sick and I realized I have nothing without my happiness. Nothing. Zero. Zilch."

CHAPTER SEVEN

Detox:
Accelerating the Change

Toxic Times

Since 1940, we have created more than 75,000 synthetic chemicals and released them into the environment and the food chain," says David Wolfe, nutritionist and superfoods and natural beauty expert. "These chemicals—from DDT to PCBs—have contaminated every single creature on earth. They are now as much a part of our bodies as oxygen and carbon. Our health has literally been under attack for years."

"The body has two ways of defending itself against these toxins," says Alejandro Junger, M.D., bestselling author of *Clean: The Revolutionary Program to Restore the Body's Natural Ability to Heal Itself*. "One is to produce mucus to coat these lipophilic, or fat-loving, chemicals so that they buffer the irritation. The second is when the body can't dissolve these chemicals, it responds by retaining or generating more fat."

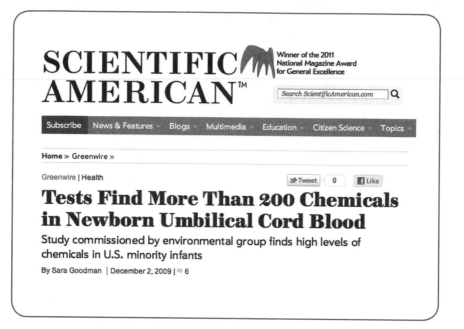

SCIENTIFIC AMERICAN™

Subscribe | News & Features | Blogs | Multimedia | Education | Citizen Science | Topics

Home » Greenwire »

Greenwire | Health

Tweet | 0 | Like

Tests Find More Than 200 Chemicals in Newborn Umbilical Cord Blood

Study commissioned by environmental group finds high levels of chemicals in U.S. minority infants

By Sara Goodman | December 2, 2009 | 6

What this means, according to Jon Gabriel, is the body won't let you get rid of this excess fat because it needs these fat deposits to protect itself against chemicals. "As long as you're taking in more toxins than you're eliminating," he says, "your body won't let you burn fat, because burning fat will release more toxins into your body, putting strain on your liver and other organs. Before your body will let you lose weight, you have to eliminate the toxins from your body. So you have to address the fact that you're being assaulted with toxins before your body will start to let go of weight."

The body only wants to take care of you. It wants to get rid of all of these chemicals in your system. "It's crying out to heal," says Jason Vale. "That's all it wants to do. It wants to naturally detoxify. Only the body can detoxify itself, provided it has the chance to do so."

We're exposed to more toxins than our bodies can handle, according to Dr. Junger. "We are experiencing a bit of an evolutionary glitch," he says. "Evolution is what happens as organisms adapt and overcome obstacles and threats. Driven by the instinct for survival, organisms learn how to transform certain chemicals into others. Over time, the human body has developed an effective and sophisticated system of organs and functions to detoxify naturally. Our physical bodies have evolved just right, but our modern lifestyle and diet prevent the body from doing what it wants to do naturally.

"As toxicity increases, our detox system should be allowed to kick in. But it can't, because it's overwhelmed by the number of toxins we take in every day. Our bodies literally can't evolve fast enough to process our modern diet. So we need to change the way we live and eat, or our bodies will shut down and die."

As David Wolfe says, "It's time to clean up. It's time to turn away from the idea of better living through chemistry and move toward the idea of better living through nature."

"A lot of us, we have some healing to do, because the world that we grew up in has been such a barrage against our nervous system and our endocrine system," says Daniel Vitalis. "Our health has been under attack. So there's going to be a period of healing."

That's the bad news. The good news is that cleansing our bodies is not complicated. In fact, it's as natural—and as important—as breathing.

> **"It's time to clean up. It's time to turn away from the idea of better living through chemistry and move toward the idea of better living through nature."**
>
> —DAVID WOLFE

The process of detoxification occurs in two steps. In step one, the liver neutralizes toxins, then expels them into the bile, which the body will later excrete through urine and sweat. And in step two, we require plenty of nutrients to rebuild healthy cells and allow our organs to function optimally.

CHLOROPHYLL

Liquid Oxygen

Found in almost all plants, chlorophyll allows plants to absorb energy from light through photosynthesis. As a powerful blood builder—and one of nature's greatest healers—chlorophyll increases red blood cell production and filters oxygen through our bodies' cellular structures, which strengthens our immune systems, improves our circulation, and cleans out harmful toxins from our livers, colons, and digestive tracts, essentially supercharging our health.

Chlorophyll-rich foods include spinach, asparagus, broccoli, kale, turnip greens, and green peppers—basically any kind of green vegetable. So just go green. For a quick chlorophyll fix, Mike Adams, the Health Ranger, suggests parsley and cilantro. "Parsley can help cleanse your entire blood supply," he says, "and it also gives you fresh breath. Parsley has so much chlorophyll that it just cleanses your whole system. Grow your own parsley, then juice it with some other vegetables and fruits to make a chlorophyll-rich, highly nutritious beverage.

"And cilantro binds with heavy metals, like mercury, a harmful neurotoxin that's often found in fish and our dental amalgam fillings. If you eat cilantro, it binds with the mercury and helps to remove it from your system."

To function properly, according to Dr. Junger, the liver needs plenty of nutrients, such as vitamin C, the B vitamins, selenium, magnesium, sulfur, and amino acids like methionine and cysteine—basically, the same nutrients and minerals found in the probiotics and superfoods discussed in chapter 3.

According to Daniel Vitalis, "Detoxing really just requires high-quality green plant food, like organic green vegetables and other foods rich in chlorophyll, which are great ways to clean out our bodies as well as rebuild the nutrients. There's some less obvious stuff, too, like gelatinous plant foods. Things like chia seeds or aloe vera or seaweed. These foods have a gel they secrete when they get wet. As they move through the intestinal tract, these gelatinous fibers absorb salts and fat-soluble toxins the liver's desperately trying to get rid of. As the liver tries to get rid of toxins, it puts it in the bile and dumps it into the small intestine, hoping that it will eventually get out of the system. Without these gelatinous fibers, the body will most likely reabsorb these harmful toxins. That's why gelatinous fibers like chia seeds are so important. You put that in your body and that can really do a lot to clean out the liver. If you combine that with the juices, the salads, the fresh young green vegetables, you've got a really great program for cleaning the body out.

"Cleansing our bodies is not complicated. Just input gentle foods, be out in nature, and our body will cleanse itself very easily."

In his bestselling book, *Clean*, Dr. Junger outlines an effective and easy-to-follow detoxification program designed to rejuvenate the body.

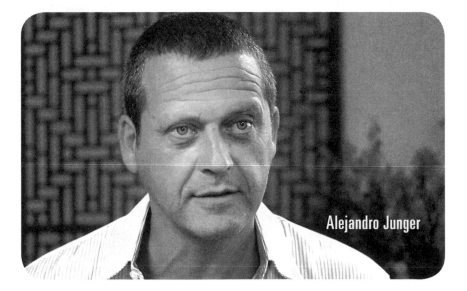

Alejandro Junger

THE *CLEAN* AUDIT

Answer the questions on this list, and note your number of "yes" answers.

Do you have headaches more than occasionally?

Do you tend to get colds or viruses each year?

Do you have bowel movements less frequently than once a day?

Do you have bowel movements that are not soft and easily passed?

Do you have diarrhea more than very rarely?

Do you get itchy or watery eyes at certain times of the year?

Do you have allergies or hay fever?

Do you often get congested or mucusy?

Do you feel bloated after eating?

Do you have extra pounds that won't come off with diet and exercise?

Do you have puffiness in areas of your face or body?

Do you have dark circles under your eyes?

Do you get heartburn?

Do you have gas more than occasionally?

Do you have bad breath or body odor?

Is there a thin white coating on the back of your tongue when you wake up?

Do you get cravings for certain kinds of foods, especially sugary, starchy, or dairy foods?

Do you have a tendency toward restless sleep?

Do you have itchy skin, pimples, or any other troubling skin condition?

Do you get pain or stiffness in your joints or muscles?

Do you have low moods or a foggy mind?

Do you find that you are forgetful, have difficulty concentrating, or can't find words?

Do you feel apathetic and tired?

Do you feel angry or have bursts of irrational frustration?

Do you have higher-than-average sensitivity to odors?

Have you noticed an increasing sensitivity to toxins in everyday life, such as feeling nauseated when you smell dry-cleaning fluid or fill up your car's tank with gas, noticing stronger effects of certain food additives, or having reactions to cleaning or personal-care products?

Do you use multiple prescription medications?

Do you have strange reactions to medications or supplements?

Do you use many potentially toxic chemicals in your home or work environment?

Do you have musculoskeletal aches and pains or symptoms suggestive of fibromyalgia?

Do you have tingling or numbness on one side?

Do you have recurrent edema?

Have you noticed a worsening of any troublesome symptoms after anesthesia or pregnancy?

If you answered "yes" to three or more of these questions, you may benefit a great deal from a short period of cleansing or detoxification, which can help to improve or clear up these symptoms and many others. For a quick and easy detox, see part III of this book. If you have many symptoms or wish to conduct a more thorough detoxification program, try the program in *Clean* by Dr. Alejandro Junger or, for a vegetarian option, in Kris Carr's *Crazy Sexy Diet*.

What Is Cleansing and Detoxification?

Cleansing is turning up the intensity and effectiveness of the detoxification system.

Cleansing and detoxification programs may be returning to popularity today, but they are certainly not new to humans. Every ancient system of health care had ways of regularly attending to the body's detoxification systems and making sure the lines of defense in the body were working properly—and this was centuries before industrial chemicals filled the air. Humans have always instinctually known that a regular period of resting and recharging the body will let it shed the accumulated toxins and waste materials that tend to build up in all of us simply from living. It is also a way to boost healing when systems are taxed and are beginning to show signs of stress.

Every creature in nature does this periodically, alternating cycles of growth and activity with cycles of rest, such as hibernation. This keeps things in balance. Animals stop consuming food when they get sick. They rest the digestive system, so that energy can be diverted toward defense and healing.

The Sanskrit word "Ayurveda" can be translated as the science of longevity. Its core philosophy is that health is a state in which the body is clear of toxins, the mind is settled, emotions are happy, wastes are constantly eliminated, and organs are working efficiently. To achieve this goal, Ayurvedic doctors give their patients balancing diets and herbs as part of a treatment plan. But they also prescribe regular periods of deeper detoxification, known as *panchakarma,* during which the patients follow a cleansing program for several weeks and have hands-on treatments to pull toxins out of tissues and quiet the busy mind. This was developed millennia before smokestacks and diesel trucks arrived on the scene. Ayurveda understands that a part of ordinary human experience is the tendency to build up waste and accumulate stress, and if we don't spend some time alleviating this at a deeper level, our systems and organs get fatigued, making us sick.

Chinese health care is similarly wise. Frequently Chinese doctors put their patients on a program of teas, tonics, and treatments to help them throw off the toxins and mental fatigue they accumulate just by eating, breathing, and meeting everyday demands. Native Americans and members of other indigenous cultures around the world have used fasting and sweat lodges to purify body, mind, and spirit. Done periodically, the sweat-lodge experience returns participants to a path of clarity on every level, or is used strategically to heal disease.

All these traditions know that the simple experience of being human brings with it the need to periodically focus on cleansing and detoxifying. When we consider the weight of our modern toxic load and its taxing effects on our inner environments, a period of detoxifying practically becomes obligatory.

It's important to distinguish between a detox program (a cleanse) and the more generalized practice of slowly "cleaning up our act" by making gradual diet or lifestyle changes over several months. A cleanse is a distinct program, done for a concentrated period of time, that puts the body in a more intense detox mode. It has a start and an end date and a specific purpose. These kinds of detoxification programs have also long been valued as a chance for the mind to come back to a peaceful center. In ancient times, cleansing through fasting was used as a tool to gain spiritual clarity. Cleaning out the amma wasn't just about diet; it was a process of cleansing the spirit of the toxic feelings and thoughts that cause suffering in the heart and soul. Jesus fasted for forty days and forty nights; Muhammad, Gandhi, and Buddha all fasted. Fasting for ultimate clarity about the nature of life is a part of many spiritual traditions and has been ingrained in humans for thousands of years.

For most people living busy lives today, the primary motivation to cleanse and detoxify is to remove the heaviness, fog, or lack of energy that is a consequence of contemporary lifestyles and stress. But dig a little deeper and there's often an underlying eagerness to simplify and strip away excess for a period of time, make some space, and get a new start by taking leave of some old, stuck patterns. There is an inevitable awakening in the mind and emotions, even if the stated goal of the cleanse is more physical, such as to enhance beauty, encourage weight loss, or look younger.

Health care in the twenty-first century is in the process of being radically reinvented. Ancient methods of protecting and preserving body and mind are being integrated with new discoveries in biochemistry and quantum physics. A new era of detox programs is being born.

(Excerpted from *Clean: The Revolutionary Program to Restore the Body's Natural Ability to Heal Itself* by Alejandro Junger, M.D., with Amely Greeven. Reprinted by permission of HarperCollins Publishers.)

If you're not ready to try a cleanse, the easiest way to accelerate your body's detoxification processes is by introducing fresh, raw, and organic plant foods into your daily diet, while making sure to get plenty of fresh air. Also, avoid industrial cleaning supplies, cosmetics, heavily perfumed soaps, or any other chemically laden products by purchasing clean alternatives. By following these simple steps, your body will respond immediately and thank you with increased energy, clarity of mind, and weight loss, letting you feel the way you've always wanted to feel.

"And when the weight starts coming off," says Daniel Vitalis, "you'll become so excited you won't want to stop. Then you'll eventually start adding more and more foods back in from healthy sources that are satisfying and nutritious. And you'll find you can live a life of not just being fit and trim but actually feeling good in a body that works properly and stays healthy forever."

Part III

GETTING STARTED

You're now ready to get started. In this section of the book, you'll find lots of great recipes, healthy lifestyle tips, menu planners, and a three-day guided detox. You'll also find recipes from the contributors in the book, our *FOOD MATTERS* team, and celebrated chef Frank Giglio—from simple and easy snacks and desserts to much more advanced culinary creations.

Remember to focus on adding in instead of eliminating. Whenever possible, ensure that your foods are as organic and natural as possible. This is about enjoying a lifelong relationship with the foods you eat.

Bon appétit.

HUNGRY FOR CHANGE
Recipes

JUICES

Super Detox Green Juice

(James and Laurentine)

SERVES 1

> 2 to 3 celery stalks, leaves removed
>
> 1 small cucumber
>
> 2 kale leaves
>
> Handful of fresh parsley
>
> 1 small lemon or lime, peeled
>
> 1 pear or apple

Juice all of the ingredients, then serve.

For an extra health kick, stir in 1 teaspoon of one or all of the following: barley grass, wheatgrass, and spirulina powder.

Super Vitality Blood Cleansing Juice

(Jon Gabriel)

SERVES 1

> **2 to 3 celery stalks, leaves removed**
> **1 large Swiss chard leaf**
> **1 carrot**
> **1 apple**
> **1 garlic clove**
> **½-inch knob of ginger root**

Juice all of the ingredients, then serve.

JUICES

Refreshing Cucumber, Pear, and Fennel Juice

(Laurentine)

SERVES 1

> **1 small cucumber**
> **2 celery stalks, leaves removed**
> **¼ fennel bulb**
> **½ lime, not peeled**
> **1 pear**

Juice all of the ingredients, then serve.

Super Simple Green Drink

(FOOD MATTERS)

SERVES 1

> **1 12-ounce glass spring or filtered water**
> **1 tablespoon barley grass or wheatgrass powder**
> **1 teaspoon spirulina powder**

Stir all of the ingredients together, then serve.

This is a highly alkalizing green drink, which helps to detoxify the blood. It may taste a little strange at first, but the more you drink it, the more you'll get used to the flavor.

Mean Green Juice

(Joe Cross)

SERVES 2

> **6 kale leaves**
> **1 cucumber**
> **4 celery stalks, leaves removed**
> **2 green apples**
> **½ lemon, peeled**
> **1-inch knob of ginger root**

Juice all of the ingredients, then serve.

▶ This is the official recipe of Joe Cross's *Fat, Sick, and Nearly Dead*.

JUICES

Ginger Lemon Detox Drink

(James and Laurentine)

SERVES 1

> **1 12-ounce spring or filtered water**
> **Juice of ½ lemon**
> **½-inch knob of ginger root**

Add the lemon juice to the glass of water. Grate the ginger finely on a chopping board, then squeeze the ginger pieces in your hand, letting the juice of the ginger drip through your fingers and into the glass of water. Enjoy at room temperature upon rising for an amazing start to the day!

Green Grape and Pear Juice

(Joe Cross)

SERVES 1

> **1 cup green grapes**
> **1 pear**
> **1 lime, peeled**
> **2 cucumbers**

Juice all of the ingredients, then serve.

Veggie Delight

(Jason Vale)

SERVES 1

4 carrots
1 apple (preferably Golden Delicious)
1 raw beet
½ lime, peeled
2 handfuls spinach leaves
1 small piece ginger root
½ zucchini

Juice all of the ingredients, then serve.

Sunshine in a Glass

(Jason Vale)

SERVES 1

> **3 carrots**
> **2 apples (preferably Gala)**
> **1 celery stalk, leaves removed**
> **½ zucchini**
> **¼ cucumber**
> **½ lemon, peeled**
> **3 broccoli florets**
> **Small handful of fresh mint leaves**

Juice all of the ingredients, then serve.

Lemon Ginger Juice

(Jason Vale)

SERVES 1

2 carrots
1 apple
½ lemon, unpeeled
¼-inch knob of ginger root
2 ice cubes

Juice all of the ingredients, then serve over ice.

Sherbet Lemonade

(Jason Vale)

SERVES 1

> **2 apples (preferably Golden Delicious)**
> **½ lemon, unpeeled**
> **2 ice cubes**

Juice all of the ingredients, then serve over ice.

Dr. Juice

(Jason Vale)

SERVES 1

> **1 small carrot**
> **2 apples (preferably Golden Delicious or Royal Gala)**
> **½ celery stalk, leaves removed**
> **1 small whole raw beet**
> **½ lemon, unpeeled**
> **½-inch knob of ginger root**

Juice all of the ingredients, then serve.

JUICES

Bruschetta Juice

(Joe Cross)

SERVES 1

2 medium tomatoes
20 fresh basil leaves
1 garlic clove

Make an incision with a knife in both tomatoes and stuff the basil leaves inside. This will help reduce the loss of leaves when juicing. Juice all of the ingredients, then serve.

Cinnamon Apple Juice

(Joe Cross)

SERVES 1

    4 cups roughly chopped butternut squash
    1 large apple (preferably Honeycrisp)
    ½ teaspoon ground cinnamon

Juice the squash and the apple, stir in the cinnamon, and serve.

Gazpacho Juice

(Joe Cross)

SERVES 1

4 plum tomatoes
1 large cucumber
2 celery stalks, leaves removed
1 red bell pepper, stemmed and seeded
¼ small red onion
2 cups fresh parsley leaves and stems, roughly chopped
1 lime, peeled

Juice all of the ingredients, then serve.

Salad in a Glass

(Jason Vale)

SERVES 1

> **1 celery stalk, leaves removed**
> **2 tomatoes**
> **¼ cucumber**
> **Handful of any type of salad greens, your choice**
> **2 carrots**
> **1 apple (preferably Golden Delicious)**
> **Handful of ice**

Juice all of the ingredients, then serve over ice.

SMOOTHIES

Turbo Charge Express Smoothie

(Jason Vale)

SERVES 1

> ¼ small pineapple, peeled
> ½ celery stalk, leaves removed
> 1-inch slice of cucumber
> Small handful of spinach leaves
> 1 lime, peeled
> 2 apples (not Granny Smiths, as they are too tart)
> Flesh of ¼ ripe avocado
> Handful of ice

Juice the pineapple, celery, cucumber, spinach, lime, and apples. Place the avocado flesh and the ice in a blender with the juiced mixture and blend for 45 seconds, or until smooth. Pour into a glass and enjoy!

For an extra health kick, add 1 teaspoon spirulina powder.

Homemade Coconut Milk

(FOOD MATTERS)

MAKES 6 CUPS

2 cups organic finely desiccated coconut (no sulfur/202/220 added)
3 cups warm spring or filtered water

Place the coconut in a blender with the water and blend for 2 to 3 minutes on high. Pour the mixture into a bowl through a fine mesh sieve lined with muslin cloth. Bring the edges together and gently strain and squeeze your milk through. Squeeze the pulp until it's dry. Use right away or keep refrigerated and sealed in a jar for up to 2 days. It will separate; just shake it and it will mix again. Reserve the leftover pulp in a zip-lock bag in the refrigerator or freezer. This can be used as coconut "flour," a great substitute for wheat flour when baking.

Homemade Nut Milk

(FOOD MATTERS)

MAKES 5 CUPS

> **1 cup raw almonds, macadamia nuts, and/or hazelnuts**
> **1 teaspoon unrefined sea salt**
> **4 cups spring or filtered water**

Put the nuts in a bowl with sea salt and enough water to cover. Cover with a plate and leave out to soak at room temperature for 4 hours or more (overnight, if desired). Drain and rinse the nuts. If running short on time, the soaking may be omitted.

Place the nuts in a blender with the water. Blend on high for about 1 minute, until it looks white and fluffy. Pour the mixture into a bowl through a fine mesh sieve lined with muslin cloth. Bring together the edges of the cloth, and drain and squeeze the milk through. Use right away or keep refrigerated and sealed in a jar for up to 2 days.

SMOOTHIES

Creamy Blueberry Smoothie

(Frank Giglio)

SERVES 1

> 1½ cups natural yogurt, raw goat milk, or desired dairy alternative
>
> 1 cup fresh or frozen blueberries
>
> 2 tablespoons chia seed gel (1 tablespoon chia seeds stirred into ¼ cup water)
>
> 1 to 2 tablespoons maple syrup
>
> 2 teaspoons spirulina powder
>
> ½ teaspoon vanilla extract or powder

Place all of the ingredients into a blender. Blend on high for 45 seconds, or until smooth and creamy.

Variations: Use fresh coconut water in place of dairy or nut milk. Add 1 tablespoon of cocoa powder for a delicious chocolate smoothie. Replace blueberries with frozen peaches, mangoes, or other seasonal berries.

Breakfast on the Move

(Jason Vale)

SERVES 1

Handful of fresh strawberries
Handful of fresh raspberries
1 cup muesli (rolled oats)
1 cup natural yogurt
1 cup milk of your choice or water
Small handful of ice

Blend all of the ingredients in a blender until smooth, then serve.

Protein Power Smoothie

(Jason Vale)

SERVES 1

> **¼ small pineapple, peeled**
> **1 apple**
> **¼ banana**
> **2 cups natural yogurt**
> **½ teaspoon spirulina powder**

Juice the pineapple and apple. Pour into a blender with the banana, yogurt, and spirulina, blend until smooth, then serve.

Spirulina Breakfast Smoothie

(Jon Gabriel)

SERVES 1

1 banana (frozen, if you prefer extra thickness)
½ cup frozen blueberries
1 medium organic free-range egg yolk
1 teaspoon spirulina
1 tablespoon ground flaxseeds
10 almonds
¾ cup yogurt or milk of choice, preferably Homemade Coconut Milk
(page 125) or Homemade Nut Milk (page 126)

Blend all of the ingredients in a blender until smooth, then serve.

Chocolate Smoothie

(Mike Adams)

SERVES 4 OR 5

> ¼ cup raw cacao nibs
> ½ cup fresh, raw coconut meat
> 1 whole avocado (seed removed)
> ¾ cup coconut milk
> ½ teaspoon stevia extract powder or 2 tablespoons raw honey
>   (sweetening this recipe is important, since cacao is naturally
>   quite bitter)
> 3 cups spring or filtered water (or until desired consistency is reached)

Blend all of the ingredients in a blender until smooth, then serve.

SMOOTHIES

Chocolate Banana Smoothie

(Jon Gabriel)

SERVES 1

> **1 banana (frozen, if you prefer extra thickness)**
> **1 tablespoon cocoa powder**
> **1 medium organic free-range egg yolk**
> **1 tablespoon ground flaxseeds**
> **1 teaspoon coconut sugar or raw honey**
> **1 cup milk of your choice, preferably Homemade Coconut Milk**
>   **(page 125) or Homemade Nut Milk (page 126)**

Blend all of the ingredients in a blender until smooth, then serve.

Strawberry Sunrise

(Jason Vale)

SERVES 1

> **¼ small pineapple, peeled**
> **1 lime, peeled**
> **½ banana**
> **4 or 5 strawberries, stemmed**
> **Handful of ice**

Juice the pineapple and lime. Pour into a blender with the banana, strawberries, and ice. Blend until smooth, then serve.

SMOOTHIES

Watermelon Crush

(Jon Gabriel)

SERVES 4

3 cups watermelon flesh, chopped
2 tablespoons lemon juice
4 to 8 whole mint leaves (optional)

Purée the watermelon flesh in a food processor or blender. Stir in the lemon juice. Place the mixture into a freezer-safe container with a lid and freeze for at least 3 hours. Remove the mixture from the freezer and let it thaw uncovered for 10 minutes before serving. Mash it with a fork, then scoop it into glasses to serve. The crush is even more refreshing when served with the fresh mint.

Piñada Colada

(Jon Gabriel)

MAKES 1 LITER

> 1 ripe pineapple, peeled, cored, and cubed
> 1 cup Homemade Coconut Milk (page 125) or canned coconut milk
> 6 tablespoons lime juice
> Ice cubes to serve

Blend all of the ingredients in a blender until smooth, then serve over ice cubes.

▶ The ripeness of your pineapple makes all the difference between a bitter and sweet piña colada!

Ginger Orange Smoothie

(Jason Vale)

SERVES 1

> **3 oranges, peeled as close to the rind as possible (the majority of nutrients are found directly under the skin)**
> **½-inch knob of ginger root, unpeeled**
> **1 banana**
> **Handful of ice**

Juice both the oranges and the ginger by placing the piece of ginger in among the oranges. Pour the orange-ginger juice into a blender, add the banana and ice, and blend until smooth, then serve.

Berry Kefir Smoothie

(James and Laurentine)

SERVES 1

> ½ cup fresh or frozen mixed berries
> 1½ cups cow or goat milk kefir or natural yogurt
> 1 teaspoon raw honey or ¼ teaspoon stevia

Blend all of the ingredients in a blender until smooth, then serve.

Strawberry and Mango Melt

(Jason Vale)

SERVES 1

> **Flesh of ½ mango**
> **Handful of strawberries, stemmed**
> **2 tablespoons natural yogurt**
> **Handful of ice**
> **Juice of 2 oranges**

Place the mango flesh, strawberries, yogurt, and ice in a blender. Pour in the orange juice and blend all until smooth, then serve.

TEAS AND HOT DRINKS

Ginger Turmeric Detox Tea

(James and Laurentine)

SERVES 1

> **1 ½ cups filtered or spring water**
> **¼ teaspoon ground ginger**
> **¼ teaspoon ground turmeric**
> **1 teaspoon maple syrup or raw honey, or ¼ teaspoon stevia**

Bring the water to a boil, then pour it into a mug. Stir in the ingredients and serve.

▶ Turmeric is an ancient Ayurvedic spice that has been used in food and medicine for centuries. It has strong anti-inflammatory properties and is also used to stimulate bowel movements.

Happy Hot Chocolate

(FOOD MATTERS)

SERVES 1

> **1 generous tablespoon raw cacao powder**
> **½ teaspoon ground cinnamon**
> **Milk of choice (nut, coconut, or organic dairy)**
> **Raw honey, coconut sugar, or stevia**

Spoon the cacao and cinnamon into a mug. Pour in boiling water straight out of the kettle until your mug is two-thirds full. Stir to combine. Then fill the remaining third of the mug with a milk of your choice and sweeten to taste. Enjoy while it's warm.

Ginger Lemon Tea

(James and Laurentine)

SERVES 1

1 cup spring or filtered water
Juice of ½ lemon, plus one slice of lemon for garnish
1-inch knob of ginger root, finely grated

Bring the water to a boil, then pour into a teacup or mug. Add lemon juice and squeeze the grated ginger in your hand as if you're making a fist, dripping the ginger juice into the mug. Garnish with a slice of lemon and enjoy!

Health Elixir Tea

(Daniel Vitalis)

SERVES 4

> 4 cups spring or filtered water
> 1 tablespoon pau d'arco bark (antifungal herb)
> 1 tablespoon passion flower tea (mood-elevating tea)
> 1 tablespoon nettle tea (cleans the kidneys and bladder)
> ½-inch knob of ginger root, finely sliced (powerful detoxifier)
> 1 tablespoon goji berries, roughly chopped (high in anti-oxidants
>   and a light sweetener)
> 2 tablespoons unsweetened coconut flakes

Place all of the ingredients in a sauce pot and bring to a boil over low heat. Reduce heat and simmer for at least 15 minutes to release the medicinal properties of the herbs into the water. Strain and enjoy warm.

Coconut Chai

(FOOD MATTERS)

SERVES 2

> 2 cups spring or filtered water
> 1 tablespoon chai spice mix (nutmeg, cloves, cardamom, cinnamon, ginger, licorice, and tea leaves)
> 1 whole piece star anise
> 2 whole green cardamom pods
> 1 teaspoon ground cinnamon
> Homemade Coconut Milk (page 125) or canned coconut milk (or nut milk, page 126, if you prefer)
> Raw honey or coconut sugar

In a sauce pot, bring the water to a boil with the chai spice mix, star anise, cardamom, and cinnamon. Then reduce the heat to low, cover, and let the spices simmer and infuse for 10 minutes. Remove from heat. Strain through a fine-mesh strainer into two mugs, until each mug is two-thirds full. Fill each mug with coconut or nut milk and sweeten to taste. Enjoy while warm.

TEAS AND HOT DRINKS

BREAKFAST

Perfect Scrambled Eggs

(FOOD MATTERS)

SERVES 1

> **2 medium organic free-range eggs, plus 1 additional egg yolk**
> **Pinch of unrefined sea salt**
> **Handful of fresh parsley, chopped**
> **1 tablespoon organic, unprocessed cultured cream or natural yogurt (optional)**
> **1 teaspoon butter**

In a bowl, whisk with some water the eggs, salt, and parsley (and the cream or yogurt, if desired). Melt the butter in a skillet set over low heat. Pour in the egg mixture and, with a spatula, gently move it around to keep it from firming up at the base and sides. When the eggs are still slightly runny, dish the mixture onto a serving plate. Let stand for a minute or two. Then serve. It works well with tomato slices, fresh or steamed greens, or cultured vegetables.

▶ Eggs, particularly the yolks, are powerhouses of nutrients rich in fat-soluble vitamins A, D, E, and K, as well as a good source of DHA, an essential fatty acid, and vitamin B12. Although it's ideal to keep yolks runny and intact, to protect the fats and proteins from denaturing, cooking eggs gently at a low temperature will protect these delicate nutrients and retain the goodness. For those who like to eat toast with their eggs, it's best to choose a fermented sourdough bread.

Veggie Frittata

(Frank Giglio)

SERVES 4

> **2 tablespoons coconut oil**
> **1 small onion, finely chopped**
> **1 red bell pepper, seeded and chopped**
> **1 small zucchini, cut in half lengthwise, then into medium dice**
> **1 large ripe tomato (½ pound), chopped**
> **¼ cup fresh parsley, roughly chopped**
> **8 medium organic free-range eggs**
> **Unrefined sea salt**
> **Freshly ground black pepper**
> **2 to 3 ounces raw goat milk cheese, grated (optional)**

Preheat the oven to 350°F.

Heat the oil in a 10- or 12-inch ovenproof skillet over medium heat. Add the onion and bell pepper, and sauté them until they begin to soften, stirring occasionally. Add the zucchini and sauté, stirring occasionally, for about 4 minutes, or until the zucchini also softens. Reduce the heat to low, add the tomato and parsley, and salt to taste. Sauté for another 3 to 5 minutes, stirring often, until the mixture begins to thicken. Taste and adjust seasonings.

In a bowl, beat the eggs until frothy and season with a ½ teaspoon of salt and pepper to taste. Pour the eggs over the vegetable mixture. Sprinkle cheese over the top, if desired. Turn the stove off and place the skillet in the oven and bake for 12 to 15 minutes, or until the eggs are set. Remove from the oven, cut into wedges, and serve.

Soft-Boiled Eggs with Asparagus

(FOOD MATTERS)

SERVES 1

> **2 organic free-range eggs**
> **3 fat asparagus spears, tough ends chopped off**
> **Unrefined sea salt**

Place the eggs (still in their shells) into a small sauce pot and cover them with cold water. Bring the pot to a boil over medium heat, then reduce the heat and simmer gently for 3 minutes. Remove from heat and hold the pot under cool running water to stop the eggs from cooking through.

In a wide skillet or frying pan, bring ½-inch of water to a simmer. Add asparagus spears and cook briefly, only until they turn bright green. Rinse them with cold water to halt their cooking process. Chop the spears in half and serve them on a plate alongside the eggs, seasoned with salt to taste. With the eggs placed either in an eggcup or on the plate, slice off one end of each egg and dip the asparagus spears into the runny yolks.

Poached Eggs over Sautéed Greens

(Frank Giglio)

SERVES 1

> **4 to 5 cups water**
> **Splash of raw apple cider vinegar**
> **1 teaspoon unrefined sea salt, plus additional for the spinach**
> **1 tablespoon coconut oil**
> **1 garlic clove, thinly sliced**
> **1 bunch spinach, well cleaned and rinsed**
> **Freshly ground black pepper**
> **2 organic free-range eggs**

Add the water to a medium sauce pot set over medium-high heat. Add the vinegar and 1 teaspoon of the salt to the water.

While you are waiting for the water to reach a simmer, heat the coconut oil in a sauté pan over medium-high heat. Add the garlic and brown without burning, then add the spinach. Stir well. Season with salt and a pinch of pepper to taste. Once the spinach is wilted, remove pan from heat and place the spinach on a serving dish.

Crack 1 egg into a small bowl, then carefully add it to the simmering water without breaking its yolk. Repeat with the second egg. Poach the eggs for 3 to 5 minutes, or as desired. Remove eggs from the water with a slotted spoon and serve them over the sautéed spinach.

Build-Your-Own Breakfast Cereal

(Frank Giglio)

SERVES 1

> ½ cup raisins (sulfur-free), soaked 20 minutes in 1 cup warm water,
> then strained
>
> 2 tablespoons chia seed gel (1 tablespoon chia seeds stirred into
> ¼ cup water)
>
> ¼ cup chopped almonds
>
> ¼ cup unsweetened coconut flakes
>
> 2 teaspoons mesquite meal (or almond or coconut meal)
>
> 6 to 8 strawberries, stemmed and quartered
>
> 1 tablespoon maple syrup

Toss all of the ingredients together in a bowl and enjoy with yogurt or milk
of your choice.

Best Bircher Muesli

(FOOD MATTERS)

SERVES 1 OR 2

> 1 cup rolled oats
> Handful of dried sour cherries, unsweetened cranberries, or currants
> Handful of unsweetened desiccated or dried coconut flakes
> 1 cup spring or filtered water
> Pinch of unrefined sea salt
> ½ cup natural yogurt or kefir
> 1 teaspoon ground cinnamon
> ½ green apple, grated
> Handful of berries of your choice
> Raw honey or pure maple syrup (optional)

In a bowl, combine the oats, dried fruit, coconut, water, and salt. Cover and let sit at room temperature for at least 12 hours, or overnight. When it's ready to serve, stir in the yogurt or kefir, cinnamon, apple, berries, and the optional honey or maple syrup, then serve. Bircher muesli keeps in the fridge for up to 5 days.

For a dairy-free version, instead of the yogurt, use ½ cup of organic apple juice to soak and then coconut milk to serve.

Homegrown Granola

(Frank Giglio)

YIELDS A LARGE BATCH, WHICH WILL KEEP FOR MONTHS

> 4 cups quick-cooking oats
> ¾ cup almonds, chopped
> ¾ cup walnuts, chopped
> 1½ cups hemp seeds
> ¾ cup chia seeds
> 1 cup raw pumpkin seeds
> 1 cup raw sunflower seeds
> 1 tablespoon ground cinnamon
> 1 teaspoon ground clove
> ¾ teaspoon ground allspice
> 1 teaspoon freshly grated nutmeg
> 2 cups grade-B maple syrup

Preheat the oven to 325°F.

Place all the ingredients except the maple syrup into a large bowl and mix thoroughly. Then stir in the syrup and coat everything well. Spread the mixture onto two large baking sheets and slowly roast in the oven until golden brown. The mixture should no longer be sticky and should feel dry to the touch. Remove from the oven and allow to cool. Store in airtight containers. The granola can be served with yogurt and/or fresh, chopped fruit.

Millet Porridge

(FOOD MATTERS)

SERVES 2

> **1 cup hulled millet**
> **Pinch of unrefined sea salt**
> **2½ cups spring or filtered water**
> **Handful of dried fruit (dates, figs, prunes, etc.)**
> **1 teaspoon ground cinnamon**
> **4 whole cardamom pods**
> **Kefir, natural yogurt, or milk of your choice**

Soak the millet in some water with the salt for 12 hours or overnight. Rinse and strain through a fine-mesh sieve, then put the millet in a sauce pot with the 2½ cups of water, dried fruit, cinnamon, and cardamom pods. Bring to a boil, then reduce to low heat and simmer, covered, until the millet is soft (about 6 minutes). Remove and discard the cardamom pods. Serve the porridge hot with kefir, yogurt, or milk.

▶ Why soak grains? In traditional cultures, grains, pulses, and nuts were mostly soaked overnight, or for many days, to prepare them for consumption. Soaking the grains and nuts activates the life-force energy within the seed and prepares it to germinate. Soaked and sprouted nuts contain more vitamins and minerals than unsoaked nuts and are more digestible.

Warm Breakfast Porridge

(Frank Giglio)

SERVES 2

> 3 cups cooked wild rice or quinoa
>
> 1 or more cups of milk of your choice or water
>
> 1 teaspoon ground cinnamon
>
> Pinch of unrefined sea salt
>
> ¼ cup toasted, unsweetened coconut flakes
>
> Maple syrup or other natural sweetener
>
> 1 tablespoon butter or coconut oil

Place the cooked rice or quinoa into a heavy-bottomed sauce pot with the milk or water, cinnamon, and salt. Gently heat, stirring the mixture often. If necessary, add more liquid. Once it's nicely hot and creamy, add the coconut, your chosen sweetener, and any additional condiments you may wish. Serve topped with a dab of butter or coconut oil.

Mushroom and Broccoli Frittata

(Dr. Joseph Mercola)

SERVES 4

> 2 cups chopped broccoli pieces
>
> 4 medium potatoes, peeled and chopped
>
> 2 teaspoons coconut oil
>
> 1 small onion, chopped
>
> 6 medium mushrooms, sliced
>
> 6 organic free-range eggs
>
> 1 cup grated cheese of your choice
>
> 1 teaspoon unrefined sea salt

Steam the broccoli and potatoes. Set aside.

Heat the coconut oil in a large skillet over medium heat. Add the onion and mushrooms and sauté together until they are soft and fragrant. Remove from heat. Add the steamed broccoli and potatoes to the skillet, stir together, and set aside.

In a large bowl, beat the eggs well, then pour them into the skillet over the vegetables. Reheat the skillet over medium-low heat and cook for about 15 minutes, or until the frittata is set but still a little moist in the middle. Sprinkle grated cheese and the salt over the top and serve. Alternately, you can cook all of the ingredients in an ovenproof skillet as instructed, then when you add the eggs, set the skillet in a preheated oven set at 350°F and bake for 12 to 15 minutes.

BREAKFAST

Nori and Eggs

(Dr. Joseph Mercola)

SERVES 4 TO 6

> 1 tablespoon toasted sesame oil
> 1 carrot, sliced into ¼-inch-thick coins
> 2 tightly packed cups spinach leaves
> 3 tablespoons wheat-free tamari
> 2 medium organic free-range eggs
> ¼ cup spinach water (see instructions)
> 4 sheets nori
> 1 teaspoon freshly squeezed lemon juice

Heat the oil in a small skillet over low heat. Add the carrot coins and sauté until soft. Remove from heat, transfer to a bowl, and let cool.

Steam the spinach until wilted. Strain and keep the strained spinach water for later use. Let the spinach cool, then squeeze it into one long, somewhat flat log shape. Sprinkle it with 2 tablespoons of the tamari.

In a bowl, whisk together the eggs, the remaining tablespoon of tamari, and ¼ cup of the reserved spinach water. Pour the egg mixture into the skillet (still with some of its oil leftover from the carrot sauté) set over medium heat. Cook the eggs as you would an omelet, eventually folding it over 4 times so that it results in one long, narrow log. Remove from heat and let cool.

Toast both sides of each nori sheet over a low burner flame or in a toaster oven, until the sheets are greenish in color. Place a toasted nori sheet on a sushi mat or a clean, flat surface. At about a half-inch from the sheet's bottom edge, place a line of carrot coins, a length of the spinach to fill the width of the nori sheet, and a section of the omelet that also fills the width of the nori sheet. Tightly roll the nori with the omelet and vegetables, keeping it firm, even, and smooth, until you have a sushi-like roll encased in nori. Using your fingers, wet the edges of the nori with lemon juice and seal it. Repeat with all of the sheets of nori and the remaining omelet and vegetables, until you have 4 rolls. Serve them as wraps or slice each roll into approximately ½-inch sushi-like pieces.

Kickin' Breakfast Burritos

(Frank Giglio)

SERVES 4

2 tablespoons coconut oil

½ small red onion, diced (roughly ½ cup)

1 red bell pepper, diced

2 teaspoons ground cumin

1 cup cooked black beans

¼ teaspoon ground cayenne or chipotle pepper

Unrefined sea salt

Freshly ground black pepper

4 medium organic free-range eggs

¼ cup milk of your choice

4 10-inch whole-wheat tortillas (or gluten-free alternative)

¼ cup tomato salsa (store-bought)

1 large tomato, diced

1 small avocado, cubed

¼ cup fresh cilantro, roughly chopped

2 to 3 ounces raw milk cheese, grated

Heat 1 tablespoon of the coconut oil in a large (at least 10-inch) skillet over medium-high heat. Lightly sauté the onions and peppers with the cumin for about 5 to 6 minutes, or until soft. Add the black beans and the ground cayenne or chipotle, and sauté for an additional 3 minutes, or until warmed through. Season with salt and pepper to taste, and transfer to a bowl or dish. Set aside.

Whisk together the eggs and milk. Heat the remaining tablespoon of coconut oil in the same large skillet over medium heat. Pour in the egg mixture and scramble for about 3 minutes, or until cooked through. After quickly warming the 4 tortillas, divide the scrambled eggs, veggie-bean mixture, salsa, tomato, avocado, and cilantro between the warmed tortillas. Sprinkle each with grated cheese, roll up burrito-style, and serve warm.

Blueberry Ricotta Pancakes

(Jon Gabriel)

MAKES 6 PANCAKES

> **4 medium organic free-range eggs**
> **4 ounces ricotta cheese**
> **¼ cup coconut flour**
> **¼ cup chia seeds**
> **1½ teaspoons coconut palm sugar**
> **½ cup blueberries, fresh or frozen**

Thoroughly whisk together the eggs, ricotta cheese, coconut flour, chia seeds, and coconut palm sugar. Gently fold in the blueberries. Lightly grease a frying pan or skillet with coconut oil, butter, or ghee and preheat to medium heat. Scoop ¼ cup batter onto the pan and flatten it out to about ½ inch thick. Brown the pancakes on both sides. They're finished when they're crispy on the outside but still a bit runny on the inside. Allowing the middle to be slightly liquid keeps the essential omega-3 oil intact. Serve with fresh fruit.

BREAKFAST

SOUPS AND STEWS

Raw Creamed Fennel Soup

(FOOD MATTERS)

SERVES 4

> 1½ cups chopped fennel (approximately 1 large bulb)
> 3 celery stalks (leaves removed)
> Flesh of 1 small to medium avocado
> ¼ cup freshly squeezed lemon juice
> ¼ cup spring or filtered water
> ½ teaspoon unrefined sea salt
> 4-inch length of green onion
> 2 ice cubes

Blend all of the ingredients in a blender until smooth, approximately
1 minute. Adjust flavors to taste. Serve garnished with fennel herb sprigs.

▶ The fennel bulb contains beneficial fibers that reduce elevated
cholesterol levels and aid in the removal of carcinogenic toxins
from the intestine.

Mineral-Rich Raw Green Soup

(Frank Giglio)

SERVES 1

> **Flesh of 1 ripe avocado**
> **1 medium tomato, cut into smaller chunks**
> **1 large handful baby spinach, well washed and drained**
> **1 small garlic clove**
> **1 green onion, roughly chopped, plus a bit more for garnish**
> **1 tablespoon fresh thyme leaves or 1 teaspoon dried thyme**
> **1 to 2 tablespoons white miso paste**
> **Freshly ground black pepper**
> **2 tablespoons cultured cream, natural yogurt, or extra-virgin olive oil**
> **Juice of ½ lemon**
> **8 to 10 ounces coconut water, filtered water, or light herbal tea (nettle, peppermint, etc.)**

Blend all of the ingredients in a high-speed blender until smooth and creamy, roughly 45 seconds. Adjust seasonings, then serve.

French Onion Soup

(Frank Giglio)

SERVES 2

> **2 tablespoons coconut oil**
> **4 yellow onions, cut in half, then thinly sliced (crescent-shape slices)**
> **1 large leek, washed well, white section cut lengthwise and then into**
>   **¼-inch-thick half-moons**
> **2 garlic cloves, minced**
> **1 bay leaf**
> **2 teaspoons dried thyme**
> **Roughly 4 cups homemade chicken and/or vegetable stock, or water**
> **Unrefined sea salt or wheat-free tamari**

Melt the oil in a large soup pot over medium-high heat. Add the onions and leeks and sauté until the mixture is golden brown in color and reduced to half its original quantity. Be mindful to keep stirring every so often to prevent burning.

Stir in the minced garlic and sauté an additional 2 minutes. Then add the bay leaf and thyme and enough stock and/or water to cover the mixture by 2 inches. Cover the pot and bring to a boil. Then immediately lower the heat and simmer slowly for 30 minutes.

Add sea salt or tamari to taste and serve.

Thai Coconut Soup

(FOOD MATTERS)

SERVES 4

> 4 cups homemade vegetable, chicken, or fish stock
> 1 teaspoon finely grated ginger root
> 1 small bunch fresh cilantro (reserve some to garnish)
> 1 stem lemongrass, cut in half lengthwise
> 3 tablespoons fish sauce (without MSG/E621) or wheat-free tamari
> Juice of 2 limes
> 1½ cups Homemade Coconut Milk (page 125) or canned coconut milk
> Wheat-free tamari or unrefined sea salt
> 1 medium-size and -heat red or green fresh chili pepper, seeded and
>   finely sliced, for garnish

In a sauce pot, bring to a boil the stock, ginger, cilantro, and lemongrass, then lower the heat and let simmer for 10 minutes. Remove from heat, discard the lemongrass, and stir in the fish sauce, lime juice, and coconut milk. Add tamari or sea salt to taste. Ladle into bowls or mugs, and garnish with chopped chili and the reserved cilantro leaves.

▶ A traditional fermented food, fish sauce is a wonderfully rich source of thyroid-nourishing iodine and is high in vitamins A and D.

SOUPS AND STEWS

Miso Soup

(Jon Gabriel)

SERVES 1

> **1 cup spring or filtered water**
> **1 tablespoon organic miso paste**
> **1 tablespoon green onions, chopped**

Boil the water and stir in the miso paste. Add the green onions, then serve.

Variation: Add cooked chicken, meat, or fish and veggies for a more substantial miso.

▶ Miso soup makes for a great light meal or satisfying quick snack. Made from soybeans, miso is a naturally fermented product with many nutritional benefits. There are many types of miso, so experiment with a few to find your favorite. Miso is also sold as a powder to be mixed with hot water. If you purchase it as a powder, check the packaging to be sure there are no added chemicals, such as MSG, artificial colors, or preservatives.

Egg and Lemon Soup with Quinoa

(FOOD MATTERS)

SERVES 2 TO 4

> **1 cup white quinoa, soaked for 12 hours in water with 1 teaspoon unrefined sea salt**
> **6 cups organic chicken or vegetable stock**
> **2 teaspoons unrefined sea salt**
> **2 organic free-range eggs**
> **Juice of 2 lemons**
> **Freshly ground black pepper**
> **Fresh dill to garnish**

Drain and rinse the soaked quinoa in a fine-mesh sieve. Then place in a large soup pot with the stock and the salt. Bring to a gentle boil. Cover and simmer over low heat until the quinoa is soft and translucent, approximately 10 minutes. Remove from heat and leave covered.

In a large bowl, whisk the eggs with the lemon juice until frothy. Whisk in one ladleful of the hot quinoa soup. Add another ladleful, whisking vigorously, followed by another, until all is incorporated gradually so as not to scramble the eggs. Then pour the entire mixture back into the pot with the remnants of the soup. Stir gently, adjust salt to taste, then serve hot with a generous grind of pepper and a sprinkle of the fresh dill.

Red Lentil and Coconut Curry Dhal

(Frank Giglio)

SERVES 4

> 2 tablespoons coconut oil
>
> 1 large onion, diced
>
> 3 garlic cloves, finely minced
>
> 3 tablespoons finely minced ginger root
>
> 1 teaspoon ground cumin
>
> 1 teaspoon ground coriander
>
> 1 teaspoon red curry paste, more or less to taste
>
> 2 cups Homemade Coconut Milk (page 125) or canned coconut milk
>
> 12 ounces tomato purée
>
> 2 cups dried red lentils
>
> 2 quarts (or more as needed) water or chicken or vegetable stock
>
> Handful of fresh cilantro (optional)

Melt the oil in a large soup pot over medium-high heat (a heavy-bottomed pot is best). Stir in the onion and sauté slowly until the onion is translucent and soft. Then stir in the garlic and ginger, cooking until fragrant. Add the cumin, coriander, and curry paste, mixing everything together well. Add the coconut milk, reduce the heat, and let the mixture simmer for 2 to 3 minutes covered before adding the tomato purée, lentils, and water or stock.

Remove the lid and simmer for roughly another 30 minutes, stirring often to keep the lentils from sticking to the pot. As the lentils cook, they will break down and thicken the soup. Add more liquid as you see fit.

When ready, add additional seasoning to taste and serve. Garnish with freshly chopped cilantro, if desired.

Instant Green Soup for One

(FOOD MATTERS)

SERVES 1

>1 tablespoon coconut oil or butter
>½ leek, dark green ends removed, and roughly chopped (or ½ onion, roughly chopped)
>1 small zucchini, roughly chopped
>1 garlic clove, minced
>Unrefined sea salt
>1½ cups spring or filtered water or homemade stock
>Large handful of baby spinach
>Handful of fresh parsley
>Juice of ½ lemon
>Freshly ground black pepper

Heat the oil or butter in a small sauce pot over medium-low heat. Sauté the leek or onion, zucchini, and garlic in the oil, salted to taste, until soft. Add the stock. Bring to a simmer, then immediately remove from heat. Stir in the spinach, parsley, and lemon juice. Put it all into a blender and blend until smooth. Add pepper and more salt to taste.

Zucchini Mushroom Soup

(Frank Giglio)

SERVES 1 OR 2

>2 tablespoons coconut oil
>6 cups roughly chopped mushrooms (crimini, portobello, or other
> wild variety)
>1 medium-size yellow onion, roughly chopped
>2 garlic cloves, chopped
>1 large zucchini, cut into ½-inch-thick half-moons
>1 bay leaf
>Purified water as needed
>2 cups of chopped cauliflower
>Unrefined sea salt
>Freshly ground black pepper
>Fresh herbs for garnish (rosemary, sage, thyme, and/or parsley)

Heat the oil in a large soup pot over medium-high heat. Sauté the mushrooms in the oil with a sprinkle of sea salt until they are lightly browned, for 3 to 4 minutes. Stir in the onion, garlic, and zucchini and cook an additional 3 to 4 minutes. Add the bay leaf and enough water to cover the vegetables. Cover the pot, bring to a gentle boil, then lower the heat to medium-low and simmer for 12 minutes. At this point, add the cauliflower and let everything continue to simmer until the cauliflower is soft.

Either purée the soup in batches in a blender or blend it with an immersion, or "stick," blender until smooth and creamy. Season to taste with salt and pepper. Serve garnished with fresh chopped herbs.

For a richer taste, stir in ¼ cup of almond milk or 2 tablespoons of coconut oil.

Raw Spinach Avocado Soup

(Frank Giglio)

SERVES 1 OR 2

> **2 cups Homemade Coconut Milk (page 125) or canned coconut milk**
> **2 ripe avocados, cut into large chunks**
> **2 handfuls baby spinach leaves**
> **¼ cup fresh cilantro**
> **Juice of 1 lime or lemon**
> **1 garlic clove**
> **2 tablespoons minced shallot**
> **Unrefined sea salt to taste**

Blend all of the ingredients in a blender until smooth and creamy. Garnish with extra cilantro leaves, extra chopped avocado, or nuts or seeds of your choice.

Mineralizing Miso Soup

(Frank Giglio)

SERVES 1 OR 2

> **3 cups warm spring or filtered water or herbal tea (nettle, horsetail, or gynostemma)**
>
> **1 long strand kelp (comes in strands when you buy it packaged), soaked in water for 20 minutes**
>
> **1 tablespoon coconut oil**
>
> **3 tablespoons chickpea miso**
>
> **Juice of 1 lemon**
>
> **10 Brazil nuts**
>
> **2 celery stalks, roughly chopped**
>
> **1 garlic clove**
>
> **2 tablespoons roughly chopped shallots**

Blend all of the ingredients in a high-speed blender for 45 seconds, or until smooth and creamy. Enjoy as is, or serve over steamed broccoli or any cooked gluten-free grain (quinoa, millet, brown rice, etc.).

Hearty Lentil Stew

(Frank Giglio)

SERVES 1 OR 2

2 tablespoons coconut oil

2 medium yellow onions, roughly chopped

2 celery stalks, cut into ½-inch chunks

2 medium carrots, cut into ½-inch chunks

2 cups dried green lentils

1 bay leaf

1 tablespoons dried Italian seasoning (a mix of basil, marjoram, oregano, rosemary, and thyme)

1 bunch of kale, chopped

1 cup frozen peas

Fresh sage, chopped

Unrefined sea salt

Freshly ground black pepper

Heat the oil in a large soup pot over medium-high heat. Sauté the onions, celery, and carrots in the oil for 3 to 4 minutes, stirring often, until they start to soften and brown. Add the lentils, stirring to coat them evenly with the oil and vegetable mixture. Add enough spring or filtered water to the pot to cover everything by an inch. Add the bay leaf and Italian seasoning. Cover the pot and bring to a boil, then reduce heat and gently simmer for 30 minutes.

Once the lentils are tender and the water is absorbed, add the kale and peas. Cook an additional 10 minutes. Stir in chopped sage to taste. Season with salt and pepper to taste, and serve warm.

SALADS AND DRESSINGS

Ruby Grapefruit, Avocado, and Fennel Salad

(FOOD MATTERS)

SERVES 2 OR 3

> 2 ruby (pink) grapefruits
> 2 avocados, sliced
> 1 large or 2 small fennel bulbs, thinly sliced
> Small handful of fresh mint leaves, torn into pieces
> 2 tablespoons extra-virgin olive oil or macadamia nut oil
> 1 tablespoon lime juice
> Unrefined sea salt
> Freshly ground black pepper

Slice the thick peel and pith from the top and bottom of the grapefruit. Thinly slice downward on all sides of the grapefruit to remove all peel and white pith and expose the grapefruit's ruby flesh. Cut segments from the flesh. Then squeeze all residual juice from the remaining core into a separate bowl. To the grapefruit segments, add the avocado, fennel, and mint.

In a glass jar or a separate bowl, shake or whisk together the olive oil, lime juice, 1 tablespoon of the remaining grapefruit juice, and a generous pinch each of salt and pepper. Pour the dressing over the salad mixture and toss gently.

Steamed Cauliflower and Broccoli with Chunky Avocado Salad

(Frank Giglio)

SERVES 2

Half a head of broccoli and/or cauliflower, cut into florets
2 ripe avocados, diced
1 small carrot, sliced into coins
½ cup chopped purple cabbage, cut into small pieces
1 garlic clove, minced
3 tablespoons fresh parsley, roughly chopped
2 tablespoons hemp seeds
½ teaspoon chili powder
2 tablespoons extra-virgin olive oil
Juice of 1 lemon
Unrefined sea salt
Freshly ground black pepper

Place the broccoli and/or cauliflower florets into a steamer basket and steam over boiling water until just fork tender. Remove from the steamer basket and arrange on two serving plates. Place the avocados into a bowl and gently toss with the carrot, cabbage, garlic, parsley, hemp seeds, chili powder, olive oil, and lemon juice. Season with salt and pepper to taste. Divide the mixture between the serving plates, placing alongside the broccoli and/or cauliflower, and enjoy.

Strawberry, Pecan, and Goat Cheese Salad

(FOOD MATTERS)

SERVES 4

> **4 handfuls mixed baby greens**
> **6 or more strawberries, stemmed and halved**
> **⅓ cup raw activated pecans (see page 239), soaked overnight**
> **2 ounces soft goat cheese**
> **⅓ cup extra-virgin olive oil**
> **2 tablespoons balsamic vinegar or raw apple cider vinegar**
> **¼ teaspoon unrefined sea salt**

Roughly tear the baby greens and arrange them in a bed on a serving platter. Scatter the strawberries, pecans, and cheese over the greens.

In a glass jar, shake together the oil, vinegar, and salt, then drizzle the dressing over the salad ingredients. Lightly toss and serve.

Blueberry Salad with Lemon Ginger Dressing

(FOOD MATTERS)

SERVES 4

For the Salad

> **Leaves from 1 bunch of fresh cilantro**
> **Leaves from 1 bunch of fresh mint**
> **Leaves from 1 bunch of fresh flat leaf parsley**
> **1 cup fresh blueberries**

For the Dressing

> **2 teaspoons finely grated ginger root**
> **⅓ cup cold-pressed macadamia nut oil, or extra-virgin olive oil**
> **Zest and juice of 1 lemon**
> **1 garlic clove, minced**
> **½ teaspoon unrefined sea salt**
> **2 teaspoons raw honey (optional)**

To prepare the dressing, first squeeze the grated ginger tightly in your hand and drip the resulting ginger juice into a glass jar. Discard the ginger pulp. In the same jar, shake together the ginger juice, oil, lemon zest, lemon juice, garlic, and salt, along with the honey (if desired).

Roughly chop the salad herbs, then toss them with the berries and the dressing. Serve immediately.

▶ Herbs are particularly dense in nutrients and high in anti-oxidants, which protect the body against cell and DNA damage.

Skin Beauty Salad

(FOOD MATTERS)

SERVES 2

> 1 small red onion, thinly sliced, ideally with a mandoline
> Juice of 3 limes
> 2 small cucumbers, sliced in half lengthwise
> 2 handfuls baby arugula
> 2 handfuls baby spinach
> 1 carrot, grated
> 2 radishes, thinly sliced, ideally with a mandoline
> Flesh of 1 avocado
> 1 tablespoon raw apple cider vinegar
> Pinch of ground cayenne pepper
> 1 teaspoon raw honey
> Handful of fresh herbs (dill, cilantro, or basil leaves)
> ¼ teaspoon unrefined sea salt

In a bowl, soak the sliced onion in the lime juice for 10 minutes. Scoop the seeds out of the cucumbers with a teaspoon and throw the seeds into a blender. Chop the cucumbers.

Arrange the arugula and spinach in a serving bowl. Top with the chopped cucumber, grated carrot, and sliced radish. Remove the onion from the lime juice and add to salad.

In the blender with the cucumber seeds, add the leftover lime juice along with the avocado, vinegar, cayenne, honey, herbs, and salt, then blend until smooth. (A dash of water helps facilitate blending.) Dollop the dressing generously on the salad and toss before serving.

▶ Onions and arugula are high in sulfur, a natural beautifying mineral that cleanses the liver and skin. Radishes and cucumbers are high in silica, which helps strengthen and moisturize hair, skin, and nails.

Big Ole Garden Salad

(Frank Giglio)

SERVES 1

For the Salad

> **2 to 3 ounces mixed greens**
> **1 red bell pepper, stemmed, seeded, and thinly sliced**
> **1 carrot, cut into half-moons**
> **1 small beet, grated**
> **Raw kernels cleaned from 1 cob of non-GMO corn**
> **6 cherry tomatoes, each cut in half**
> **2 tablespoons chopped chives**
> **2 to 3 tablespoons raw sunflower seeds**
> **¼ cup dulse flakes**

For the Dressing

> **Flesh of 1 ripe avocado**
> **1 medium garlic clove**
> **¾ to 1 cup spring or filtered water**
> **¼ cup raw apple cider vinegar**
> **2 teaspoons raw honey**
> **2 teaspoons Mexican spice blend**
> **4 cups thinly sliced cabbage**

To make the dressing, blend all of the dressing ingredients in a blender at high speed until smooth and creamy. Add water as needed to reach desired consistency. Any leftover dressing can be stored in the fridge for up to four days.

Place all the salad ingredients in a large bowl. Drizzle with the dressing and mix to coat everything well. Toss in some salt to taste, then serve.

Caesar Salad Dressing

(Jon Gabriel)

MAKES ¾ CUP

> 1 medium organic free-range egg yolk
> 2 teaspoons Dijon mustard
> 1 garlic clove
> 2 tablespoons lemon juice
> 3 anchovies
> ¼ cup Parmesan cheese
> ½ cup extra-virgin olive oil

Combine the egg yolk, mustard, garlic, lemon juice, anchovies, and Parmesan in a food processor. Add the oil gradually until you achieve a smooth and creamy consistency. Drizzle over your salad, sprinkle with flaxseeds, and serve.

Mayonnaise

(Jon Gabriel)

MAKES ¾ CUP

> **2 medium organic free-range egg yolks**
> **1 teaspoon Dijon mustard**
> **1 tablespoon white wine vinegar**
> **1 tablespoon lemon juice**
> **½ cup extra-virgin olive oil**
> **Unrefined sea salt and black pepper to taste**

Combine the egg yolks, mustard, vinegar, and lemon juice in a food processor or blender. Gradually add the oil in batches, whisking the mixture until well combined before adding more. Once all the oil has been added, mix for a few more seconds to achieve a thick and creamy consistency. Add the salt and pepper to taste. The mayonnaise can be refrigerated for up to 2 days.

Honey Mustard Dressing

(Jon Gabriel)

MAKES ¾ CUP

1 teaspoon grain mustard
1 teaspoon raw honey
2 tablespoons white wine vinegar
½ cup extra-virgin olive oil
Unrefined sea salt and pepper to taste
1 tablespoon parsley (optional)

Place the mustard, honey, vinegar, oil, salt, and pepper in a jar. Screw the lid on tightly and shake to combine. Pour the dressing on a salad just before serving or place the dressing jar on the table for people to use on their own. Garnish the salad with the parsley.

Niçoise Salad Dressing

(Jon Gabriel)

MAKES ¾ CUP

> 1 tablespoon ground flaxseeds
> 1 green onion, finely chopped
> 1 garlic clove, minced
> 1 teaspoon Dijon mustard
> 1 tablespoon white wine vinegar
> 1 tablespoon lemon juice
> ⅔ cup extra-virgin olive oil
> ¼ cup basil leaves
> Unrefined sea salt and pepper to taste

Blend all the ingredients except the salt and pepper in a blender until the mixture is well combined. Season to taste with the salt and pepper.

Celery, Bitter Greens, and Egg Salad with Anchovy

(FOOD MATTERS)

SERVES 2 TO 4

For the Salad

> **4 medium organic free-range eggs**
> **2 handfuls endive, roughly chopped**
> **2 handfuls baby romaine leaves, roughly torn**
> **2 celery stalks, leaves removed, finely sliced**

For the Dressing

> **Leaves from 2 young rosemary sprigs, finely chopped**
> **1 garlic clove, finely chopped**
> **8 anchovy fillets, tinned or bottled in olive oil, drained and chopped**
> **Juice of 1 lemon**
> **¼ cup extra-virgin olive oil**

Boil the eggs in water for 3 to 4 minutes, then rinse them under cool water. Set aside.

Arrange the endive and romaine salad leaves with the sliced celery on a serving platter.

In a glass jar, vigorously shake together all of the dressing ingredients. Pour enough dressing over the salad leaves and celery to coat everything well when tossed. Peel and chop the eggs and sprinkle them over the top. Gently toss the salad again. The egg yolks will add thickness to the dressing.

Roasted Vegetable Salad with Yogurt Dressing

(FOOD MATTERS)

SERVES 2 TO 4

For the Salad

1 cup sweet potato or yam, roughly chopped into ½-inch cubes

1 cup pumpkin or butternut squash, roughly chopped into ½-inch cubes

1 fresh beet, roughly chopped into ½ inch cubes

2 small yellow onions, quartered

1 zucchini, chopped into 1-inch pieces

2 tablespoons coconut oil

½ teaspoon unrefined sea salt

1 teaspoon ground cumin

¼ teaspoon ground turmeric

4 handfuls mixed tender leafy greens (arugula, romaine, baby spinach, etc.)

1 handful fresh herbs (mint, cilantro, or flat leaf parsley), roughly chopped

For the Dressing

½ cup natural yogurt

2 tablespoons extra-virgin olive oil

1 garlic clove, minced

Unrefined sea salt

Preheat the oven to 340°F.

On a large baking tray, spread the sweet potato or yam, pumpkin or squash, beet, onions, and zucchini. Drizzle the vegetables with the coconut oil, tossing to coat all sides, and sprinkle with the salt, cumin, and turmeric. If your coconut oil is hard, heat it for a few minutes in the oven on the baking tray before adding the vegetables and spices, then toss the vegetables in the oil on the tray. Roast the vegetables for approximately 20 minutes, then to make sure they are cooked evenly, toss them on the tray, and return them to the oven to roast for another 25 minutes, or until they are golden and soft to the touch. When the vegetables are ready, remove them from the oven and let cool.

In a glass jar, shake together all of the dressing ingredients. Arrange the greens and fresh herbs on a large serving dish. Toss the roasted vegetables in with the greens and herbs, then drizzle dressing over everything and serve.

Asian-Inspired Quinoa Salad

(Frank Giglio)

SERVES 2 TO 4

> **1½ cups quinoa**
> **1 tablespoon ground turmeric**
> **1 cup arame (common Japanese seaweed), soaked for 20 minutes, strained and rinsed**
> **1 cup grated carrots**
> **¾ cup thinly sliced rounds of zucchini**
> **1 red bell pepper, seeded and stemmed, cut into medium-size chunks**
> **¼ cup fresh cilantro, roughly chopped**
> **¼ cup sesame seeds, toasted**

For the Dressing

> **1 tablespoon minced ginger root**
> **⅛ cup extra-virgin olive oil**
> **¼ cup ume plum vinegar**
> **Wheat-free tamari**

Before preparing this recipe, it is quite beneficial (but optional) to soak and sprout the quinoa.* To do so, soak the quinoa in a bowl in 3 cups of water. Let it sit at room temperature for 2 hours, then strain and rinse well. Return the strained quinoa to a bowl and let it sit at room temperature for another 8 to 12 hours. You should see little tails shooting out of each little quinoa seed. Rinse again. In a sauce pot, bring 2¾ cups of water to a boil, then add the quinoa. Cover and simmer over medium heat for a total of 10 minutes, but around 5 minutes into the cooking, add the turmeric to the water. Once done cooking, turn off the heat and let sit, covered, for 5 minutes before emptying the quinoa into a bowl.

While the cooked quinoa is still warm, stir in the arame, carrots, zucchini, bell pepper, cilantro, and sesame seeds.

To make the dressing, gently whisk all of the dressing ingredients until well incorporated. Stir enough dressing into the quinoa mixture to evenly coat everything, then serve.

*If time is running short, bring 3 cups of water to a boil in a sauce pot, then pour in the quinoa and lower the heat. Simmer covered for 12 to 15 minutes. Repeat the same final steps as described above, adding the turmeric and letting it cool.

Arugula, Parmesan, and Pomegranate Salad

(FOOD MATTERS)

SERVES 2 OR 3

> 1 large ripe pomegranate
> 2 handfuls young arugula or spinach leaves
> 2 tablespoons extra-virgin olive oil
> 1 tablespoon raw apple cider vinegar
> Pinch of unrefined sea salt
> Freshly cracked black pepper
> 1½ ounces raw parmesan, shaved

To extract the seeds and juice of the pomegranate, cut the pomegranate in half. Hold a cut side down in your palm and, over a wide bowl, whack a wooden spoon against the back of the pomegranate. Seeds and juice should strain through your fingers. Scoop out any remaining pits with a spoon. Repeat with the other half of the pomegranate. Then strain the juice from the seeds, into a glass jar.

Arrange the arugula or spinach greens on a serving platter. In the jar containing the strained pomegranate juice, add the oil, vinegar, salt, and a grind of pepper, then shake vigorously. Drizzle the dressing over the greens, then scatter pomegranate seeds and parmesan shavings over the top. Serve.

Chinese Salmon Salad

(Frank Giglio)

SERVES 2

For the Salad

> **8 ounces wild salmon fillet**
> **2 cups shredded Napa cabbage**
> **1 cup fresh spicy greens (watercress, mustard, etc.), torn into bite-size pieces**
> **1 large carrot, julienned**
> **3 or 4 radishes, very thinly sliced**
> **¼ cup fresh cilantro, roughly chopped**
> **1 tablespoon sesame seeds**

For the Dressing

> **3 tablespoons brown rice vinegar**
> **2 tablespoons toasted sesame oil**
> **2 tablespoons extra-virgin olive oil**
> **1 tablespoon freshly grated ginger root**
> **1 tablespoon chickpea miso**
> **Pinch of red chili powder**

Preheat the oven to 350°F.

In a large bowl, whisk together all of the dressing ingredients. Place the salmon fillet in a baking dish and coat the fillet on all sides with a few spoonfuls of the dressing. Bake the fish uncovered for 10 to 12 minutes, then remove from the oven and let cool.

Flake the salmon into a large bowl. Add the cabbage, spicy greens, carrot, radishes, cilantro, and sesame seeds. Gently toss everything with any remaining dressing until all is evenly coated, then serve.

Warm Avocado Chicken Salad

(Jason Vale)

SERVES 2

> **2 skinless chicken breasts (preferably free-range and organic)**
> **2 handfuls of arugula**
> **1 large ripe avocado**
> **2 ounces raw Parmesan cheese**
> **Juice of 1 lemon**
> **Extra-virgin olive oil**

Grill the chicken for 20 minutes or until cooked through. Then cut into generous chunks.

Wash the arugula and place in a salad bowl. Chop the avocado, also into generous chunks, and add along with the chicken to the salad. Using a peeler or a sharp knife, shave thin slices of Parmesan over the top. Pour the lemon juice over everything, along with a healthy drizzle of olive oil.

Scrumptious Burger Salad with Lemon-Herb Vinaigrette

(Frank Giglio)

SERVES 1

For the Burger

> **4 ounces grass-fed ground beef, venison, or bison**
> **2 teaspoons freshly chopped thyme (or dried thyme)**
> **1 clove garlic, freshly minced**
> **1 teaspoon unrefined sea salt**
> **Pinch of freshly ground black pepper**
> **1 tablespoon coconut oil**

For the Salad

> **2 ounces fresh salad greens**
> **1 small tomato, cut into chunks**
> **8 to 10 green beans, blanched**
>
> **½ cup broccoli florets, steamed**
> **¼ cup pitted kalamata olives**
> **A few thin slices of red onion**

For the Lemon-Herb Vinaigrette

> **¼ cup raw apple cider vinegar**
> **½ to ¾ cup extra-virgin olive oil**
> **1 garlic clove, minced**
> **½ teaspoon dried oregano**
>
> **1 tablespoon whole grain mustard**
> **2 teaspoons raw honey (optional)**
> **Pinch of unrefined sea salt**
> **Freshly ground black pepper to taste**

To make the burger, mix the thyme, garlic, salt, and pepper with the ground meat, then form into a patty. Melt the coconut oil in a heavy-bottomed skillet over medium-high heat. Carefully place the burger into the skillet. Cook about 2 to 3 minutes on each side, or to desired temperature.

While the burger is cooking, prepare the salad and the vinaigrette. The vinaigrette can be made by whisking together all of the vinaigrette ingredients or, alternately, by placing them all into a jar and shaking vigorously. In a bowl, toss all of the salad ingredients—the greens, tomato, green beans, broccoli, olives, and onion—with enough of the vinaigrette to coat everything evenly. Then form the salad into a pile on a serving plate. Once the burger is cooked, place it directly on top of the salad, or chop it up and toss everything together.

Gorgeous Greek Salad

(Jason Vale)

SERVES 2

> **5 ounces goat cheese**
> **½ red onion**
> **½ red pepper**
> **½ yellow pepper**
> **¼ cucumber**
> **Large handful of plump, pitted kalamata olives**
>   **(or other olives of your choice)**
> **Handful of baby tomatoes**
> **Extra-virgin olive oil**
> **Balsamic vinegar**
> **Freshly ground black pepper**

Cut the goat cheese, onion, peppers, and cucumber all into generous chunks and place them into a salad bowl. Add the olives and tomatoes and stir together thoroughly. Add a generous splash of olive oil and balsamic vinegar over the salad. Season with black pepper to taste.

Quinoa Salad with Fragrant Spices

(Frank Giglio)

SERVES 2 OR 3

1½ cups quinoa
1 tablespoon ground turmeric
1 crisp apple, cut into small chunks
3 celery stalks, cut into thin half-moons
1 small red onion, minced
½ cup fresh cilantro, roughly chopped
½ cup fresh parsley, roughly chopped
3 tablespoons extra-virgin olive oil
1 to 2 tablespoons raw apple cider vinegar
1 tablespoon whole cumin seeds, toasted
1 teaspoon ground coriander seeds
Unrefined sea salt
¼ cup raw pumpkin seeds
¼ cup pomegranate seeds (if available)

Before preparing this recipe, it is quite beneficial (but optional) to soak and sprout the quinoa.* To do so, soak the quinoa in a bowl in 3 cups of water. Let it sit at room temperature for 2 hours, then strain and rinse well. Return the strained quinoa to a bowl and let it sit at room temperature for another 8 to 12 hours. You should see little tails shooting out of each little quinoa seed. Rinse again. In a sauce pot, bring 2¾ cups of water to a boil, then add the quinoa. Cover and simmer over medium heat for a total of 10 minutes, but around 5 minutes into the cooking, add the turmeric to the water. Once done cooking, turn off the heat and let sit, covered, for 5 minutes before emptying the quinoa into a bowl. Cool to room temperature.

Once the quinoa has fully cooled, stir in the apple, celery, onion, cilantro, and parsley. Stir in the olive oil and apple cider vinegar. Season with the cumin and coriander, and a touch of sea salt, as desired. Garnish with pumpkin seeds and pomegranate seeds, if available.

To bulk up this dish, add cooked chickpeas, or serve with grilled chicken or freshly roasted wild-caught fish, such as salmon, haddock, or halibut.

*If time is running short, bring 3 cups of water to a boil in a sauce pot, then pour in the quinoa and lower the heat. Simmer covered for 12 to 15 minutes. Repeat the same final steps as described above, adding the turmeric and letting it cool.

Cauliflower Mash

(FOOD MATTERS)

SERVES 2 TO 4 AS A SIDE

> **1 head cauliflower, trimmed and cut into florets**
> **1 tablespoon butter**
> **1 garlic clove, finely chopped**
> **½ teaspoon unrefined sea salt**
> **¼ teaspoon freshly ground black pepper**
> **Ground nutmeg (if fresh, use a fine grater or microplane)**

Put the cauliflower florets into a steamer basket set over boiling water. Steam until tender. Transfer to a colander to let excess liquid drain.

Combine the cauliflower, butter, garlic, salt, and pepper. You could either mash everything with a potato masher in a bowl or put everything through a food processor. Adjust seasoning to taste. Serve sprinkled lightly with nutmeg.

▶ Cruciferous vegetables like cauliflower are lower in starch (carbohydrates) and far higher in nutrients than potatoes. Other low-starch vegetables that mash well without the glycemic load include kohlrabi and celeriac. The addition of butter (from grass-fed cows) adds vital fat-soluble nutrients that facilitate the absorption of minerals and other fat-soluble nutrients.

Spinach Rice

(FOOD MATTERS)

SERVES 4 TO 6

> 2 tablespoons butter or coconut oil
> 1 large leek, white section only, finely sliced
> 2 garlic cloves, finely chopped
> 1 cup basmati rice
> 2 cups hot water or homemade stock
> 2 small bunches organic spinach, well washed
> Handful of fresh dill, chopped
> Handful of fresh parsley, chopped
> 2 tablespoons freshly squeezed lemon juice
> Unrefined sea salt
> Freshly ground black pepper
> Extra-virgin olive oil

Melt the butter in a large, deep sauce pot over low heat. Sauté the leek and garlic in the butter until they are soft and aromatic. Add the rice and stir well to fully coat the grains with the butter and leeks. Add the water or stock plus ½ teaspoon of sea salt, and bring to a gentle simmer. Let it simmer, covered, over low heat for 10 to 15 minutes, or until the liquid is absorbed and the rice is cooked, adding more liquid as needed so it doesn't burn. Remove from heat and leave the mixture to stand, covered.

Cut any woody stalks off the spinach leaves, rinse well, and put the leaves into a pot of simmering water ½-inch deep. Cover for just a minute or two, to allow the leaves just to wilt. Drain, then squeeze out the excess liquid.

Chop the spinach roughly, then add it along with the dill, parsley, and lemon juice to the rice mixture. Salt and pepper to taste. Serve drizzled with the olive oil and garnished with extra lemon wedges, if desired.

▶ Basmati is a long-grain, fragrant rice with a lower glycemic index than other rice varieties. This is due to its high amylose content, a type of carbohydrate more resistant to digestion, so there is less of an effect on blood sugar levels.

Wilted Kale

(FOOD MATTERS)

SERVES 4

> **1 bunch of organic kale of any variety, such as purple or curly**
> **1 or 2 lemons**
> **Unrefined sea salt**
> **Cultured butter or extra-virgin olive oil**

Remove the woody stems of the kale with a knife or scissors. Wash the leaves with filtered water, leaving them wet. Put the leaves in a pot set over medium heat. When the kale just reaches a simmer, reduce the heat to low, cover, and cook for 6 to 8 minutes, or until the leaves have completely wilted and are bright green.

Strain the kale in a colander and squeeze out any excess liquid by pushing with the back of a spoon. Chop the kale roughly and place on a serving dish. While still warm, squeeze a generous amount of lemon juice over the top, sprinkle with salt, and top with a knob of butter or a drizzle of olive oil.

Raw, Dairy-Free Zucchini Alfredo

(FOOD MATTERS)

SERVES 4

4 zucchini
1 cup raw macadamia nuts, soaked overnight in water
   with 1 teaspoon salt
1 garlic clove, crushed
1 cup extra-virgin olive oil
½ cup spring or filtered water
Juice of 1 lemon
2 teaspoons wheat-free tamari
¼ teaspoon ground cayenne pepper
Pinch of unrefined sea salt

Note: This dish tastes just like pasta Alfredo without being too heavy or rich.

Peel the zucchini thinly with a vegetable peeler, so that they resemble fettuccini ribbons.

Blend together in a blender all of the remaining ingredients—the nuts, garlic, oil, water, lemon juice, tamari, cayenne, and salt—and pour over the zucchini ribbons as your sauce.

Veggie Fritters

(Jon Gabriel)

MAKES 6

> **2 tablespoons extra-virgin coconut oil**
> **1 small brown onion, diced**
> **⅓ cup broccoli, finely chopped**
> **1 clove garlic, crushed**
> **1 medium organic free-range egg**
> **⅓ cup carrot, grated**
> **⅓ cup zucchini, grated**
> **1 teaspoon thyme**
> **Unrefined sea salt and pepper to taste**

Heat 1 tablespoon of the coconut oil in a frying pan on medium heat. Place the onion, broccoli, and garlic in the frying pan and cook for approximately 3 minutes. Remove the pan from the heat.

Beat the egg in a medium bowl. Transfer the onion, broccoli, and garlic from the frying pan to the bowl. Add the carrot, zucchini, thyme, and salt and pepper. Mix until well combined and everything is coated in egg.

Wipe the frying pan clean with a paper towel. Heat just enough coconut oil in the frying pan to prevent sticking, then place dessert-spoon-size scoops of the mixture into the frying pan. Scoop from the bottom of the bowl to be sure you are getting egg in your scoop. Cook 2 minutes on each side or until lightly browned. Between batches, wipe the frying pan clean and reapply cooking oil. Serve the fritters sprinkled with flaxseeds.

Sweet Potato Fries

(FOOD MATTERS)

SERVES 3 OR 4

> **2 medium sweet potatoes, peeled and cut into ½-inch-thick fries**
> **3 or 4 tablespoons coconut oil**
> **Unrefined sea salt**
> **Mild or sweet ground paprika**

Preheat the oven to 410°F.

Line a baking sheet with parchment paper. Toss sweet potato fries on the tray with coconut oil to coat (melt the oil first, if necessary). Arrange the fries so they are not overcrowded on the tray. Sprinkle generously with salt and dust with paprika.

Bake for 10 minutes. Remove from oven, turn each piece over and return to oven. Bake for another 10 to 15 minutes, until golden on the outside and soft in the middle.

▶ Baked in coconut oil and devoid of trans fats, this makes a nutritious and tastier alternative to the usual. Try making fries out of other root vegetables, such as parsnips, celeriac, or carrots.

Asian-Style Green Beans

(Dr. Joseph Mercola)

SERVES 6

> **1 tablespoon coconut oil**
> **1 pound green beans trimmed and cut into 2-inch pieces**
> **2 garlic cloves, minced**
> **2-inch knob of ginger root, minced**
> **3 tablespoons wheat-free tamari**
> **¼ cup freshly squeezed lemon juice**
> **Unrefined sea salt**
> **Freshly ground black pepper**
> **Raw sesame seeds**

Heat the oil in a heavy-bottomed sauté pan over medium-high heat. Sauté the green beans in the oil for 2 minutes. Add the garlic, ginger, and tamari, and continue to sauté until the beans are tender-crisp, approximately 4 minutes. Remove from heat and toss with lemon juice. Add salt and pepper to taste. Serve sprinkled with sesame seeds.

Garlic Spiced Collard Greens

(Dr. Joseph Mercola)

SERVES 5

> **1 large bunch collard greens (approximately 1½ pounds)**
> **2 tablespoons coconut oil**
> **1 medium garlic clove, chopped**
> **½ teaspoon dried chili flakes**
> **Unrefined sea salt**
> **Freshly ground black pepper**
> **Juice of 1 lemon**
> **Feta cheese**

Wash the greens thoroughly under running water and pat dry. Remove the stems and cut the greens into 1-inch strips. Heat the oil in a large sauté pan over medium-high heat. Sauté the garlic in the oil until it just begins to brown, about 30 seconds, then add the collard greens and chili flakes. Cook only until the greens wilt. Add salt and pepper to taste, and remove from heat. Toss with the lemon juice and serve sprinkled with feta cheese.

Hijiki-Shiitake Sauté

(Dr. Joseph Mercola)

SERVES 4

> **1 cup hijiki (a seaweed found in Asian stores)**
> **3 cups spring or filtered water**
> **1 medium onion, sliced**
> **1 carrot, sliced into matchsticks**
> **1 tablespoon toasted sesame oil**
> **2 cups shiitake mushrooms, sliced**
> **1 cup apple juice**
> **2 tablespoons wheat-free tamari**
> **1 teaspoon freshly grated ginger root**

Soak the hijiki for 10 minutes in water. Strain and keep the water.

In a sauce pot, sauté the onion and carrot in sesame oil until the onion is transparent. Add the hijiki, the hijiki soaking water, the shiitakes, and the apple juice. Cover and bring to a boil, then lower the heat and simmer gently for 45 minutes.

Stir in the tamari and juice squeezed from the grated ginger. Simmer until most of the liquid is evaporated, about 15 minutes. Serve warm or chilled.

Ginger Baby Bok Choy

(Dr. Joseph Mercola)

SERVES 4

> **6 heads baby bok choy**
> **1½ tablespoons seasoned rice vinegar**
> **1½ tablespoons wheat-free tamari**
> **1 tablespoon mirin**
> **½ teaspoon raw honey**
> **2 tablespoons toasted sesame oil**
> **1 tablespoon coconut oil**
> **Pinch of red pepper flakes**
> **3 garlic cloves, minced**
> **1 tablespoon freshly minced ginger root**
> **2 green onions, sliced**
> **1 teaspoon freshly squeezed lemon juice**
> **1 tablespoon toasted sesame seeds**

Note: Have all ingredients ready, as the stir-frying is rather quick.

Cut the bottoms off the bok choy heads. Separate the leaves and cut them into small pieces, keeping the stems and leaves separate.

In a bowl, whisk together the vinegar, tamari, mirin, honey, and sesame oil, then set aside.

Warm a sauté pan or wok over high heat. Add the coconut oil, making sure to coat all areas of the pan. Stir-fry the bok choy stems with the red pepper flakes, garlic, ginger, and green onions for 30 seconds. Add the sauce mixture and stir-fry for about another minute, until the mixture thickens. Add the bok choy leaves and stir-fry another 30 seconds, until the leaves are wilted. Remove to a serving bowl, drizzle with lemon juice, and sprinkle with sesame seeds. Serve immediately.

Sweet and Sour Brussels Sprouts

(Dr. Joseph Mercola)

SERVES 4 TO 6

> **1 pound Brussels sprouts, ends trimmed**
> **2 tablespoons balsamic vinegar**
> **2 tablespoons maple syrup**
> **1 teaspoon Dijon mustard**
> **2 tablespoons olive oil**
> **½ cup roasted peanuts**
> **Unrefined sea salt to taste**
> **Freshly ground black pepper to taste**

Boil the Brussels sprouts in a medium sauce pot of salted water for 7 minutes, or until tender. Drain and cut them into quarters.

In a bowl, whisk together the vinegar, maple syrup, and mustard, then slowly drizzle in the olive oil, whisking until it's fully emulsified.

Combine the Brussels sprouts, peanuts, salt, and pepper. Pour the vinaigrette over the top and toss to coat. Serve immediately.

VEGETABLE DISHES

Roasted Tempeh with Shiitake and Sweet Potato

(Frank Giglio)

SERVES 2

1 12-ounce block organic, non-GMO tempeh, cut into 4 equal pieces

For the Marinade

2 garlic cloves
2 tablespoons whole grain mustard
2 tablespoons raw honey or maple syrup
2 tablespoons balsamic vinegar
2 tablespoons raw apple cider vinegar
½ cup extra-virgin olive oil

For the Shiitake and Sweet Potato

2 tablespoons coconut oil
1 sweet potato, washed (and peeled, if desired), cut into ½-inch dice
1 medium red onion, cut into ½-inch dice
8 to 10 shiitake mushrooms, stems removed
2 garlic cloves, minced
4 kale leaves, stems removed, torn into bite-size pieces
Unrefined sea salt

To prepare the tempeh, place the cut pieces into a non-reactive glass baking dish. Blend all of the marinade ingredients together in a blender for 30 seconds, then pour over the tempeh. Allow tempeh to marinate for at least 1 hour or, ideally, overnight.

Preheat the oven to 350°F.

Bake the marinated tempeh in its baking dish for 30 minutes. Tempeh is baked sitting in its marinade. While the tempeh is baking, make the hash. Melt the oil in a heavy-bottomed pan, preferably cast-iron, over medium-high heat. When the oil is hot, add the sweet potato and onion. Sauté, stirring often to prevent sticking, until the sweet potatoes are just about fork tender. Stir in the shiitake caps, garlic, and kale leaves. Sauté all until the kale is wilted and tender. Season with salt to taste, then divide the mixture between two serving plates. Top with pieces of the baked tempeh and serve.

Omelet Pizza

(Jon Gabriel)

MAKES 1

> 1 tablespoon butter or coconut oil
> 4 medium organic free-range eggs, beaten
> 2 tablespoons tomato pizza sauce
> 8 baby spinach leaves
> 1 mushroom, sliced thinly
> ¼ medium yellow onion, sliced thinly
> ¼ cup cheddar cheese, grated
> ¼ cup mozzarella cheese, grated

Preheat the oven to 350°F.

Heat the butter in a medium-size frying pan on medium heat. Pour the eggs into the pan. Swirl the pan to evenly distribute the eggs and cook until the underside is cooked through, about 1 minute. Reduce the heat and flip the omelet over to cook the second side. Take caution when flipping to avoid breaking the omelet. Cook until the omelet is cooked through, about another minute.

Remove the omelet and place it on a plate or wooden cutting board. Spread the tomato sauce evenly over the omelet. Add the spinach, mushroom, onion, and cheeses.

Place the prepared omelet pizza in the oven for a few minutes, until the cheese has browned.

▶ By using an egg base you introduce protein into your meal rather than dead carbs, without sacrificing taste. Use homemade sauce if you have it. Otherwise, feel free to use a store-bought sauce. When choosing, however, make sure to go with one that has organic tomatoes, no sugar or artificial sweeteners, or at the very least, no artificial colors or flavors. The other component to a great pizza is toppings, so choose all the fresh, healthy, yummy toppings you like.

Greens with Almond and Lemon

(Jon Gabriel)

SERVES 8

2 teaspoons butter or coconut oil, melted

1 teaspoon lemon rind, grated

1 tablespoon lemon juice

¼ cup almonds, blanched and sliced

2 bunches broccolini

2 bunches asparagus

1 handful sugar snap peas

Place the butter, lemon rind, and lemon juice in a glass jar. Screw on the lid tightly and shake to combine. Lightly toast the almonds in a dry frying pan over medium heat. Lightly steam the broccolini, asparagus, and sugar snap peas for 1 minute or until they are bright green in color. Place the steamed greens in a serving dish. Top the greens with the almonds and drizzle with the lemon mixture, then serve.

FISH, SEAFOOD, AND MEAT

Hemp Pesto Halibut

(Frank Giglio)

SERVES 4

>1 medium beet, finely diced (equal to roughly 1 cup)
>1 garlic clove, diced
>½ cup hemp seeds
>Juice of 2 lemons, plus thin lemon slices as needed
>½ cup fresh basil leaves
>¼ cup extra-virgin olive oil, plus additional for the fish
>1 pound halibut, cut into 4 fillets (or any wild-caught fish,
>   such as cod or haddock)
>1 to 2 teaspoons unrefined sea salt
>Freshly ground black pepper
>2 large handfuls of lettuce greens tossed in a mix of olive oil and
>   lemon juice

Preheat the oven 350°F.

To prepare the pesto, place the beet, garlic, and hemp seeds into a food processor. Pulse until finely chopped, then add the lemon juice and basil, plus salt to taste. Keep processing while drizzling in the olive oil. This pesto is best on the thicker side, so only add enough oil to help purée the mixture. Purée to the smooth consistency of a typical pesto, then set aside.

To prepare the fish, coat the fillets with olive oil, salt, and pepper. Place them in an oiled baking dish, covering each fillet with thin slices of lemon. Bake uncovered for 10 to 25 minutes, or until the fillets are cooked through (check with a fork).

To serve, divide the lettuce greens between four serving plates. Top each bed of greens with a baked fillet, then place a scoop of the pesto onto each piece of fish. Serve warm.

Steamed Bass with Fennel, Parsley, and Capers

(Frank Giglio)

SERVES 2

> **¼ medium white onion, sliced**
> **1 fennel bulb, thinly sliced**
> **Juice of ½ lemon**
> **2 5-ounce portions of striped bass**
> **½ teaspoon unrefined sea salt**
> **1 tablespoon capers, rinsed**
> **¼ cup fresh parsley, chopped**
> **Extra-virgin olive oil (for garnish)**
> **Chopped fresh parsley (for garnish)**

Put the onion, fennel, and lemon juice in a medium sauce pot and cover with one inch of water. Bring to a boil, then lower the heat slightly and simmer for 5 minutes. Remove from heat and place the 2 portions of fish into the pot. Season with salt, and sprinkle with capers and parsley. Cover the pot and simmer for about 8 to 10 minutes, or until the fish is almost flaky.

Divide the vegetables between two shallow serving bowls. Top each serving with the fish. Drizzle with olive oil and sprinkle with chopped fresh parsley. If desired, serve with steamed brown rice.

Asian-Flavored Tuna with Stir-Fried Vegetables

(Frank Giglio)

SERVES 2

½ cup nama shoyu or wheat-free tamari

1-inch knob of ginger root, thinly sliced

2 garlic cloves, crushed

2 teaspoons brown rice syrup or coconut nectar

10 ounces tuna or yellowtail, cut into 1-inch chunks (a white fish
can also be substituted, such as striped bass or cod)

1 tablespoon extra-virgin olive oil

1 teaspoon sesame oil

1 carrot, sliced on the diagonal

1 cup chopped broccoli, cut small

1 zucchini, sliced on the diagonal

1 head baby bok choy, sliced lengthwise

In a bowl, whisk together the nama shoyu or tamari, ginger, garlic, and the rice syrup or coconut nectar. Place the tuna chunks in the mixture and let marinate for a few minutes.

Set your broiler to high. Divide the marinated tuna chunks evenly between 2 grilling skewers. Broil the tuna skewers for 1 to 2 minutes, turn them over and broil another 1 to 2 minutes on their opposite sides. Set aside.

Heat the olive and sesame oils together in a sauté pan over high heat. Add the carrot, broccoli, and zucchini, and stir to coat everything with oil. Continue stirring as the vegetables cook for 2 minutes. Add the bok choy plus ¼ cup of water. Cover the pot for 1 minute, allowing the vegetables to steam slightly. Remove from heat.

To serve, place the vegetables in a flat bowl and top with the tuna skewers. Serve hot.

Provençal Snapper with Swiss Chard

(Frank Giglio)

SERVES 2

> 2 6-ounce fillets of snapper, pin bones removed
> Grated zest from one lemon
> ¼ cup capers
> 2 sprigs fresh thyme (plus more for garnish, if desired)
> Extra-virgin olive oil to drizzle over the fish,
>   plus 1 tablespoon for the chard
> Unrefined sea salt
> Freshly ground black pepper
> 4 cups of Swiss chard, washed and roughly chopped

Preheat the oven to 425°F.

In an oiled baking dish, place the snapper fillets. Sprinkle them with the lemon zest and capers, and lay the thyme sprigs over the top. Drizzle with the olive oil and season with salt and pepper to taste. Cover the dish with foil. Bake for 15 minutes.

While the fish is baking, heat the 1 tablespoon of olive oil in a sauté pan. Add the Swiss chard, cover, and let the chard steam for just 2 minutes.

Serve the fish on a bed of the chard. Spoon any remaining baking juices and capers over the fish. Garnish with additional sprigs of fresh thyme.

Wild Salmon Collard Wraps

(Frank Giglio)

SERVES 2

> 8 to 10 ounces wild-caught salmon, cut into 6 even strips
> 3 large collard green leaves
> 2 nori sheets, each sheet cut into 8 rectangles
> 1 carrot, thinly sliced
> 1 small fennel bulb, thinly sliced
> Fresh cilantro leaves for garnish
> Handful of sunflower sprouts for garnish

For the Marinade

> ¼ cup sesame oil
> ⅛ cup brown rice vinegar
> 1 tablespoon whole grain mustard
> 1½ tablespoons wheat-free tamari
> 1 garlic clove, minced
> 1-inch piece of ginger root, minced

To make the marinade, whisk together the oil, vinegar, mustard, and tamari. Then whisk in the minced garlic and ginger. Place the strips of salmon into the bowl of marinade, turning them to coat. Marinate for 20 to 30 minutes.

To prepare the collard wraps, first cut the tougher stems from the leaves of the collard greens. This will give you 2 separate pieces per leaf. Lay each leaf piece onto your work surface, dark/shiny side down. Place 1 or 2 cut nori sheet rectangles in the middle of each leaf. Place 1 marinated salmon strip on the nori, top with some carrots, fennel, cilantro leaves, and sprouts. Drizzle some of the remaining marinade over everything. Roll each collard leaf with your hand to form a roll that is open at both sides.

Optional: Place the salmon collard rolls in a bamboo steamer or a steamer basket set over simmering water and steam for approximately 5 to 6 minutes. Serve on their own or with rice and lime wedges.

Wild Salmon Ceviche with Coriander and Lime

(FOOD MATTERS)

SERVES 4

> 1 pound wild-caught salmon fillets, skinned, deboned,
>   sliced into ½-inch-thick pieces
> Juice of 4 limes
> 1 small red onion, finely chopped
> 2 garlic cloves, finely chopped or crushed
> 2 small fresh red medium-heat chili peppers,
>   deseeded and finely chopped
> 2 tablespoon chopped fresh cilantro leaves, plus more for garnish
> Unrefined sea salt
> Freshly ground black pepper

Place the salmon pieces in a large, non-metallic bowl. Stir together the lime juice, onion, garlic, chili peppers, and cilantro, and pour over the fish. Cover and refrigerate, letting the fish marinate for at least 4 hours. (Lime or lemon juice is so powerfully acidic, it more or less "cooks" the fish.)

Serve the fish (drained of all excess liquid) garnished with more chopped cilantro. Salt and pepper to taste.

Alternatively, drizzle the fish with coconut milk and serve on top of fresh salad greens. Leftovers are good the next day.

▶ Salmon is best when wild-caught and uncooked. The delicate essential fatty acid omega-3, common in salmon, is particularly heat sensitive and easily damaged by any temperature above a gentle simmer or poach. True wild salmon (the open-water dwelling, river-running species) is not only high in anti-aging, anti-inflammatory omega-3 but is also a source of quality protein, vitamins D, B12, B6, and powerful anti-oxidants such as selenium

Curry-Spiced Fish Cakes with Mango Salsa

(Frank Giglio)

SERVES 2

> 2 cups mackerel meat (haddock or other white fish will work well too)
> 1 tablespoon freshly grated ginger root
> ¼ cup roughly chopped fresh cilantro
> 1 dried or fresh red chili pepper, chopped finely (any red chili pepper of high heat)
> 1 heaping tablespoon mixed curry spice powder
> 1 tablespoon unrefined sea salt
> 1 medium organic free-range egg
> 2 tablespoons sprouted wheat or coconut flour (or sourdough breadcrumbs)
> 1 tablespoon coconut oil or ghee for cooking

For the Mango Salsa

> 1 ripe mango, chopped into medium dice
> ½ teaspoon dried or fresh red chili pepper
> ¼ cup minced red onion
> 2 tablespoons freshly chopped cilantro
> Juice of 1 lime

To prepare the salsa, gently toss all of the salsa ingredients in a bowl, then let sit at room temperature for 20 to 30 minutes.

To prepare the fish cakes, heat the coconut oil in a frying pan and cook the fish on medium high heat on both sides until tender and the flesh becomes white and flaky. Let the fish cool and place it into a food processor. Pulse it into small pieces, but avoid over-processing; it is nice to have some texture in the cakes. Place the processed fish into a bowl, add the ginger, cilantro, chili pepper, curry spices, and sea salt. Mix well. Stir in the egg, then the flour. Form equal portions of the mixture into cakes of desired dimensions.

Heat the coconut oil or ghee in a skillet over medium heat. Brown each side of the fish cakes, continuing to cook them until they are hot all the way through. Remove from the pan and serve with the mango salsa and possibly with a mix of fresh greens.

Steamed Fish in Lemon and Herbs

(FOOD MATTERS)

SERVES 1

> **1 7-ounce fillet of thick, firm, white, non-oily fish (snapper, trout,**
> **sea bass, cod, halibut, sole, turbot, whiting, or wild barramundi)**
> **3 green onions, roots and dark green ends removed, sliced into**
> **1-inch lengths**
> **2 lemon slices, plus an extra lemon wedge for the garnish**
> **1 tablespoon butter or coconut oil**
> **1 teaspoon fish sauce (no MSG/E621)**
> **Pinch of unrefined sea salt**
> **Handful of fresh cilantro, finely chopped (reserve some for the**
> **garnish)**

Preheat the oven to 230°F.

Cut a piece of parchment paper roughly 20 inches long. Place the fish fillet in the center and top it with the green onions, lemon slices, butter or coconut oil, fish sauce, and salt. Bring the long ends of the paper together and fold down securely several times, then fold down or twist the ends tightly and fold the ends under the fish. You should have a tightly wrapped packet of your fish. Bake for 45 minutes or until just cooked.

The fish should easily flake, by this point. Open the parcel and serve immediately, with all of its cooking juices, garnished with the lemon wedge and a sprinkling of cilantro leaves.

For more of a Mediterranean flavor, swap the cilantro for basil or parsley, and add to the bag things like halved cherry tomatoes, crushed garlic, raw black olives, fennel, and/or basil leaves.

For more of an Asian-inspired flavor, add to the bag grated ginger root, chopped fresh or dried flakes of hot chili pepper, chopped lemongrass, tamari, and/or a couple of tablespoons of coconut cream. Garnish with a wedge of lime and fresh mint.

▶ Cilantro is a powerful and natural detoxifying herb that works to remove mercury and other heavy metals from the blood and brain.

James's Mom's Fijian Fish Curry

(FOOD MATTERS)

SERVES 4

1 tablespoon coconut oil

1 medium yellow onion, finely chopped

2 garlic cloves, chopped

1 teaspoon zest of unwaxed lime (reserve lime juice for garnish)

2 tablespoons ground garam masala spice blend

1 teaspoon ground turmeric

2 teaspoons ground sweet paprika

1 teaspoon ground cumin

Half a bunch of fresh cilantro, roots and stems chopped,
     leaves reserved for garnish

½ cup water

1 tablespoon tamarind paste, dissolved in a small amount of
     warm water (stir or strain any lumpy bits and discard)

1 teaspoon unrefined sea salt

2 pounds mahimahi or similar firm wild-caught whitefish,
     diced into 1-inch pieces

1 cup coconut milk

1 medium-hot, fresh green chili, deseeded and finely chopped
     for garnish

Heat the oil in a large sauté pan over low heat. Add the onions and garlic, and sauté gently until the onions are translucent. Add the lime zest, garam masala, turmeric, paprika, cumin, and cilantro roots and stems. Sauté, stirring constantly, for about 2 minutes or until fragrant. Then add the water, tamarind, and salt and heat everything until it's just barely simmering.

Place the pieces of fish into the pan and poach until they are almost cooked through, stirring gently so as not to break them up. Remove the pan from heat and add the coconut milk, stirring gently for another minute. Serve immediately, garnished with chopped chili, the fresh cilantro leaves, and a generous squeeze of fresh lime juice.

Sesame Encrusted Salmon with Coconut Kale

(Dr. Joseph Mercola)

SERVES 4 TO 6

For the Salmon

> **6 salmon steaks**
> **4 tablespoons butter**
> **4 tablespoons coconut oil**
> **4 tablespoons minced ginger root**
> **1 cup raw sesame seeds**

For the Kale

> **3 tablespoons coconut oil**
> **2 tablespoons minced ginger root**
> **1 bunch kale, chopped**
> **1½ cups coconut milk**
> **Unrefined sea salt**
> **Freshly ground black pepper**

To prepare the salmon, melt the butter and oil together with the ginger (perhaps in a small sauté pan set over low heat). Brush the butter, oil, and ginger mixture on all sides of each salmon steak, then roll the steaks in the sesame seeds, coating them completely. Place the salmon steaks on an oiled baking sheet and refrigerate them for about 15 minutes.

Preheat the oven to 475°F.

While the salmon is in the fridge, prepare the kale. Heat the oil in a large skillet over medium heat, then sauté the ginger for 3 minutes. Add the kale and sauté, stirring constantly, for another 5 minutes. Add the coconut milk and season to taste with salt and pepper. Bring the mixture to a boil, cover, and slightly reduce the heat. Simmer until the kale is tender. Set aside.

Take the baking sheet of salmon steaks from the refrigerator and place it into the preheated oven. Roast the salmon until the sesame seeds are golden brown yet the salmon is still rare inside, 3 to 5 minutes. Season to taste with salt and pepper, and serve immediately alongside a helping of the kale.

Shrimp and Kale Sauté

(Frank Giglio)

SERVES 2

> **6 cups water**
> **1 teaspoon unrefined sea salt**
> **1 head broccoli, cut into florets**
> **2 cups kale, roughly chopped**
> **1 tablespoon coconut oil**
> **¼ cup sliced yellow onion**
> **2 celery stalks**
> **2 garlic cloves, sliced**
> **1 pound shrimp, peeled and deveined**
> **Juice of 1 lemon**
> **1 tablespoon natural lemon pepper seasoning (or use your own homemade mix of lemon zest and cracked peppercorns)**
> **3 cups steamed wild rice**

In a medium to large pot, heat the water, salted to taste, and keep it just under a boil. Blanch the broccoli florets in the water for 2 to 3 minutes, or just until tender. Set the florets in a colander, and rinse them with cold water to immediately halt the cooking. Set aside. Repeat the same steps with the kale.

Heat the oil in a large cast-iron or stainless-steel sauté pan over medium-high heat. Lightly sauté the onion, celery, and garlic in the oil for 1 to 2 minutes. Add the shrimp and gently toss. Continue to sauté, tossing gently, for another 2 to 3 minutes, or until the shrimp are about halfway cooked through. Toss in the broccoli and the kale, then add the lemon juice and lemon pepper, plus a splash of additional water. Cover the pan and let cook for another 3 to 5 minutes. Adjust seasonings and add unrefined sea salt to taste. Serve immediately over steamed wild rice.

Chili Garlic Ginger Shrimp

(Dr. Joseph Mercola)

SERVES 4

> ¼ cup coconut oil
> 2-inch knob of ginger root, minced
> 2 cloves garlic, minced
> 2 small fresh medium-heat red chilies, deseeded and thinly sliced
> 16 large shrimp (approximately 1 pound), peeled and deveined
> Juice of 1 to 2 lemons
> ½ cup fresh flat leaf parsley, roughly chopped
> Unrefined sea salt
> Freshly ground black pepper

Heat the oil in a large sauté pan over medium-high heat. Add the ginger, garlic, chilies, and shrimp. Sauté for about 3 minutes, stirring often.

Turn down the heat to low, and stir in the juice of 1 lemon and the parsley. Remove from heat. Salt and pepper to taste and add more lemon juice, if desired. Serve immediately. The shrimp goes well with steamed rice or on a bed of steamed greens.

Lemon Scallops with Parsley

(Dr. Joseph Mercola)

SERVES 4

> 1 tablespoon coconut oil
>
> 2 pounds sea scallops, cut into pieces
>
> ¾ teaspoon unrefined sea salt
>
> ½ teaspoon freshly ground black pepper
>
> 1 tablespoon butter
>
> 1 teaspoon minced fresh garlic
>
> ¼ cup finely minced shallots
>
> ⅓ cup dry white wine
>
> 2 tablespoons freshly squeezed lemon juice
>
> 1 tablespoon chopped fresh flat leaf parsley

Heat the oil in a large sauté pan over medium-high heat. Add the scallop pieces and sprinkle with salt and pepper. Sauté the scallops 2 minutes on each side. Remove the scallop pieces from the pan and set aside.

In the same pan, melt the butter. Sauté the scallop pieces approximately 2 minutes, or until each side is lightly seared. Add the garlic and shallots, and sauté for about 1 minute. Add the wine and sauté for another 2 minutes. Return the scallops to the pan and toss them to fully coat. Then remove the pan from the heat.

Serve the scallops garnished with sprinkles of lemon juice and chopped parsley.

Chili Mussels

(Jon Gabriel)

SERVES 4

> 2 pounds mussels
> 1 tablespoon butter or coconut oil
> 1 medium yellow onion, diced
> 1 garlic clove, peeled and chopped
> 2 cups tomatoes, puréed
> 1 teaspoon chili powder or fresh chili, or to taste
> ½ cup fresh basil leaves, finely shredded

Rinse and debeard all the mussels. Discard any open mussels that do not close when held under running water while applying pressure. Set aside. Heat the butter in a medium sauce pot on medium heat. Add the onion and sauté until it begins to color. Add the garlic and allow it to cook for 1 minute. Add the tomatoes and chili powder. Stir until the sauce is well heated, then remove it from the heat. Place the mussels in a large, empty pot on high heat. Heat the mussels covered for approximately 5 minutes or until they open. Place them in one large serving bowl or divide among four individual serving bowls. Distribute the sauce over the mussels. Stir and sprinkle with shredded basil leaves before serving.

Slow-Cooked Grass-Fed Beef Osso Buco

(FOOD MATTERS)

SERVES 4

1 tablespoon butter
2 yellow onions, finely chopped
2 celery stalks, finely chopped
2 carrots, finely chopped
3 garlic cloves, chopped
2 teaspoons unrefined sea salt
8 anchovies, bottled in olive oil or brine, drained
4 bay leaves
1 whole cinnamon stick, snapped in half
2 fresh thyme sprigs or 1 teaspoon dried thyme
¾ cup red or dry white wine (organic, sulfur-free,
   or containing minimal sulfur: 220/202)
4 ripe tomatoes or 1 cup tomato purée out of a glass bottle
½ cup spring or filtered water
4 or 5 shank cuts of grass-fed and -finished beef osso buco
½ teaspoon freshly ground black pepper
Fresh flat leaf parsley, chopped, for garnish

Preheat the oven to 195°F.

Melt the butter in a large cast-iron pot set over low heat. Add the onions, celery, carrots, garlic, and salt, and gently sauté until everything is soft and the onions are translucent. Add the anchovies, mashing them into the base of the pot with the back of a wooden spoon until the anchovies begin to melt. If you omit them, add more of the unrefined sea salt.

Add the bay leaves, cinnamon stick pieces, and thyme, and pour in the wine. Increase the heat slightly and gently simmer everything for another couple of minutes. The alcohol will cook out and the liquid will reduce slightly. Then add the tomatoes, the water, and the pepper, stirring thoroughly to incorporate, and remove the pot from heat.

Gently add the beef pieces and submerge them in the liquid and vegetables until they are positioned at the bottom of the mixture. Cover and place in the oven. Cook for 10 to 12 hours. (For a quicker cooking time, set the oven to 250°F. It will be ready in 6 to 8 hours.)

The osso buco is ready when it's tender and easily comes away from the bone. Serve with its nutrient-rich sauce spooned over each piece and a generous sprinkling of chopped of parsley as a garnish. If desired, pair the osso buco with a simple green salad, or sauerkraut to aid digestion. And don't forget to eat the marrow!

▶ This is a particularly nutrient-dense meal. When cooked at such a low temperature, the meat is more tender, the nutrients are retained, the proteins are undamaged, and the fats are protected from oxidation. Cooking meats on the bone adds additional minerals and gelatin to the dish. We recommend using beef rather than veal, for ethical reasons, and meat that is grass-fed and -finished, from cows raised more naturally, grazing on open pastures in full sunlight.

FISH, SEAFOOD, AND MEAT

Slow-Roasted Spiced Organic Chicken

(FOOD MATTERS)

SERVES 4

> 2 garlic cloves, crushed
>
> 2 teaspoons dried oregano
>
> 1 teaspoon ground sweet paprika
>
> ½ teaspoon ground cayenne pepper
>
> 1 teaspoon unrefined sea salt
>
> 1 large unwaxed lemon, quartered
>
> 1 whole organic, free-range chicken (approximately 4 pounds)
>
> Homemade stock or spring water
>
> Assorted vegetables for slow-roasting, such as peeled whole shallots, any type of winter squash cut into 2-inch chunks, wedges of fennel bulb, whole garlic cloves, or any other vegetables of your choice

Preheat the oven to 250°F.

In a small bowl, mix together the garlic, oregano, paprika, cayenne, salt, and 1 tablespoon of lemon juice squeezed from the lemon wedges. Rub the mix all over the outside and inside of the bird. Stuff the lemon quarters inside the bird's cavity, then place the bird breast-side up in a large roasting pan. Add vegetables around it and pour in enough stock or water to reach approximately 1-inch deep around the chicken.

Cut a piece of parchment paper large enough to fit fully around the rim of your pot while stretching the paper over the chicken. Put the lid on, securing the parchment paper between the pot and the rim. This will help keep the chicken moist. Place the pan in the oven. Slow-roast for at least 3 hours.

Remove the lid (not the paper), and cook for another 30 to 60 minutes. (If you like, at this point you can remove the parchment paper and turn the temperature up to 275°F, which will help crisp and color the skin. Otherwise leave the temperature at 250°F.)

Depending on the size of the bird, it will be ready when a leg pulls away easily and the juices are clear. Lift the chicken out of the pot and spoon out the vegetables. Reserve the cooking juices to drizzle over the chicken when serving. Any remaining cooking liquid can be kept refrigerated for use as a broth or a base for soups and other stews.

Serve the chicken surrounded by the roasted vegetables, perhaps with a fresh salad or cultured vegetables. It keeps in the refrigerator for up to a week. Freeze for longer storage.

▶ The ideal way to cook a pasture-raised organic chicken is long and slow, and at a low temperature so as not to oxidize its delicate fatty acids. The addition of liquid (stock or water) in the pot helps keep the meat tender and easily digestible. In general, limit chicken consumption to once or twice a week, favoring ruminants (grass-eating animals) and wild-caught fish, both of which have better fatty acid ratios. Chicken, even organic, has quite a high omega-6 to -3 ratio. Also, never buy "corn-fed" birds. As with any meat, always only purchase naturally raised and fed poultry, ideally from a local farmer.

FISH, SEAFOOD, AND MEAT

Slow-Cooked Chicken Thighs

(Frank Giglio)

SERVES 2

> 4 thighs from organic, pasture-raised chickens (skin on)
> 1 teaspoon unrefined sea salt, plus additional for final seasoning
> ½ teaspoon freshly ground black pepper
> 1 teaspoon ground fennel seed
> 2 tablespoons coconut oil
> 2 garlic cloves, minced
> 3 ounces (approximately ⅓ cup) white wine
> 8 ounces tomato purée
> 2 cups chicken stock
> 1 fennel bulb, quartered
> 1 cup chopped zucchini, cut into ½-inch chunks
> 1 tablespoon chopped fresh or 1 teaspoon dried thyme
> Freshly squeezed lemon juice (optional)

Allow the chicken thighs to come to room temperature, then season each with the 1 teaspoon salt, the pepper, and the fennel seed.

Melt the oil in a large skillet over medium-high heat. Add the chicken, skin side down. Cook for 5 to 8 minutes, allowing the skin to become nice and brown. Then flip the chicken and stir in the garlic, cooking until fragrant. Pour in the white wine: When the wine is reduced by half, add the tomato purée and the chicken stock. Cover and simmer for 10 minutes. Add the fennel bulb and zucchini and continue to simmer, covered, for another 15 minutes.

To finish, sprinkle in the fresh thyme, season with additional sea salt, and perhaps a splash of lemon juice, if desired. Serve as is or possibly over roasted potatoes, steamed rice, or cooked quinoa.

Chili

(Jon Gabriel)

SERVES 4

> 1 tablespoon coconut oil
> 1 medium yellow onion, sliced
> 1 pound ground meat
> 1 medium green bell pepper, cut into small pieces
> 4 tomatoes, crushed, or 1 14.5-ounce can tomatoes
> 2 tablespoons tomato paste
> 1 clove garlic, peeled and chopped
> Juice from ½ lemon
> ¼ cup red wine
> ½ teaspoon cumin
> ½ teaspoon chili powder, or to taste
> Unrefined sea salt and pepper to taste

Heat the coconut oil in a large frying pan on medium heat. Add the onion and cook it until lightly browned. Add the ground meat, stirring to separate. Stir in the bell pepper, tomatoes, tomato paste, and garlic. When the meat is cooked through, add the lemon juice, wine, cumin, and chili powder. Stir to combine. Season with salt and pepper, and serve.

SNACKS AND DESSERTS

Avocado with Raw Apple Cider Vinegar

(James and Laurentine)

SERVES 1

> **1 ripe avocado**
> **1 tablespoon raw apple cider vinegar**
> **1 tablespoon extra-virgin olive oil**
> **Pinch of unrefined sea salt**

Cut the avocado in half and remove the pit. Pour the apple cider vinegar and olive oil into the holes where the pit once was. Garnish with sea salt. Eat in its peel, scooping out the seasoned flesh with a spoon.

Variation: You can mix a bit of natural Dijon mustard and freshly ground black pepper in with the oil and vinegar.

Kale Chips

(FOOD MATTERS)

SERVES 2 OR 3

> 1 bunch curly kale
> 1 tablespoon extra-virgin olive oil
> 1 garlic clove, crushed
> ½ teaspoon unrefined sea salt
> Ground paprika, ground cayenne pepper, or chili flakes,
>   if you like a bit of heat (optional)

Preheat the oven to 170°F.

Rinse the kale leaves and dry well, patting them down with a towel (or use a dehydrator if you have one). Slice out the woody inner stems of the leaves and discard (or reserve the stems to add possibly to a soup broth, if desired). Tear or cut the remaining leaves into large pieces. In a large bowl, toss the leaves with a mix of the olive oil, garlic, and salt, plus any of the optional items, if desired. Make sure all of the leaves are fully coated.

Arrange the pieces in a single layer (not overlapping) on two large baking sheets lined with parchment paper. Bake for about 2 hours, or until the "chips" are crisp. Serve after they've slightly or fully cooled.

Variation: Try making chips out of root vegetables, such as parsnips, celeriac, or carrots.

▶ Don't eat excessive amounts of raw or dehydrated kale if you have thyroid issues. Kale, like all in the cabbage family, can block the uptake of iodine to the thyroid.

Sourdough Buckwheat Savory Crêpes or Fluffy Pancakes

(FOOD MATTERS)

SERVES 4

This recipe is based on traditional fermentation methods used to produce naturally leavened savory flatbreads. We've included two variations: One results in a savory crêpe while the other uses eggs for a fluffy sweet pancake. Fermentation time normally takes one to two days, so plan ahead!

> **1 cup whole buckwheat**
> **Spring or filtered water**
> **Unrefined sea salt**
> **1 teaspoon whey (the liquid off the top of yogurt)**

Put the buckwheat in a bowl with 2 cups of water and a pinch of salt. Cover with a plate or towel, and leave to soak at room temperature for at least 9 hours, or up to 24 hours. Then rinse the buckwheat in a fine-mesh sieve to remove the slime and residual tannins.

Put the buckwheat in a blender with another good pinch of salt, ⅓ to ½ cup of water (or enough to get a consistency similar to pancake batter), and whey (if desired). Blend until smooth. Pour the batter into a clean bowl and let stand, covered, for another 12 to 24 hours in order to form cultures. The mixture may rise a little as the good bacteria do their thing.

Once it's fermented, the mixture can be stored in a refrigerator in a glass bowl covered with a damp tea towel or plastic wrap until needed, but keep no longer than four days.

Savory Buckwheat Crêpes

For simple savory buckwheat crêpes, you can use the mixture as is.

Melt some coconut oil or butter in a skillet over medium heat. When the skillet is hot, pour in a ladleful of the batter, then tilt to allow the batter to spread over the entire bottom of the pan. When the crêpe is cooked almost all the way through, flip it to brown the other side. These work great as a gluten-free bread alternative, or sweeten them with jam or honey and yogurt.

Fluffy Buckwheat Pancakes

> **1 organic free-range egg, lightly beaten**
> **½ cup unprocessed milk, nut milk, coconut milk, or spring water**
> **1 teaspoon pure vanilla powder or natural vanilla extract**
> **2 additional organic free-range egg whites, whisked to form
>   stiff peaks**
> **Coconut oil or butter**

For fluffy, sweet buckwheat pancakes, begin with the base batter, then add the egg, milk or water, and vanilla. Mix thoroughly. Then fold in the stiff egg whites, gently incorporating them until well combined but still light.

Melt the coconut oil or butter in a skillet over medium heat. When the skillet is hot, pour in half a ladle of the batter. When the pancake is cooked almost all the way through, flip it to brown the other side.

▶ Buckwheat is in the same family as sorrel (a green leafy herb) and rhubarb. It is the seed of the plant, not actually a grain, and contains no gluten. When properly prepared by soaking, sprouting, and fermenting, as it was in traditional cooking, buckwheat's natural phytase goes to work to make it easily digestible, nutritious, and not irritating to the gut.

Buckwheat Sesame Crackers

(FOOD MATTERS)

YIELDS 20

> **1 cup buckwheat flour**
> **3 tablespoons raw sesame seeds**
> **¼ teaspoon unrefined sea salt**
> **1 tablespoon whey (the liquid off the top of yogurt; or additional salt, if whey is unavailable)**
> **¾ cup spring or filtered water**
> **¼ cup organic arrowroot powder**
> **2 tablespoons coconut oil or butter, melted, plus extra for oiling the parchment paper or foil**

In a bowl, mix together the flour, sesame seeds, salt, whey, and water. Cover and leave in a warm place for 12 to 24 hours.

Preheat the oven to 390°F.

Add to the batter the arrowroot powder (a thickening agent) and the 2 tablespoons of oil or melted butter. Combine well. The dough should be thick enough to form into a ball.

On your work surface, spread 4 large pieces of waxed or parchment paper cut to identical sizes and each approximately the size of a baking sheet. Lightly oil one side of each piece with coconut oil or melted butter. Place half of the ball of dough in the center of one sheet, then place a second oiled sheet, oiled side down (next to the dough), over the first, sandwiching the dough between the two sheets. Repeat with the third and fourth pieces of paper and the remaining half of the dough, creating, in the end, two "sandwiches."

With a rolling pin or the side of a wine bottle, roll the dough between the sheets into a very thin, perhaps ⅛-inch-thick cracker. Then carefully peel back the top sheet of paper or foil and discard it.

With a knife, slice vertical and horizontal lines through the dough, about 2 inches wide, to create cracker shapes. Lift each square onto a baking sheet and sprinkle with sea salt to your taste.

Place the baking sheet in the oven. Immediately lower the oven's temperature to 355°F. Bake for 12 to 15 minutes, or until the rows of crackers sitting closest to the edges of the baking sheet appear golden and crispy.

Remove the sheet from the oven, and lift off the outer rows of crackers, placing them on a wire rack to cool. (Cooking time will be determined by how thinly you've rolled your dough.) Separate the remaining squares with a spatula or carefully pull them apart with your hands. Turn the oven off and put the rest of the crackers back into the oven for another 10 to 20 minutes until they've dried to your liking. Once they too have fully cooled on a wire rack, transfer all of the crackers to an airtight container and store them in a pantry or fridge.

Baked Stuffed Apples

(FOOD MATTERS)

SERVES 4

> **4 unwaxed Granny Smith apples**
> **Zest of ½ unwaxed lemon**
> **¼ cup almond or macadamia nut meal, or finely chopped Activated**
> **Nuts (see page 239) (use up pulp from making Nut Milk; page 126)**
> **2½ ounces soft cultured butter or coconut oil**
> **8 dates, pitted and finely chopped**
> **½ teaspoon natural vanilla extract**
> **½ teaspoon ground cinnamon**
> **1 tablespoon raw cacao powder (optional)**

Preheat the oven to 250°F.

Carefully cut into the top of each apple and scoop out its core with a teaspoon, creating a hollow cavity while also keeping the whole of each apple intact, in order to hold the stuffing.

To prepare the stuffing, combine in a bowl the lemon zest, nut meal, butter or oil, dates, vanilla, cinnamon, and optional cacao powder. Rub everything in the bowl together with your fingertips to incorporate well.

Fill the cavity of each apple with the stuffing mixture, then set the apples on a parchment-lined baking sheet. Bake for up to 1 hour, or until soft. Serve immediately, while still hot.

Variation: Try this recipe with nectarines, peaches, or plums, or any other larger in-season fruit.

Chocolate Seed Treats

(Jon Gabriel)

MAKES 10

⅓ cup almonds
1 tablespoon sunflower seeds
1 tablespoon pumpkin seeds
1 tablespoon organic desiccated coconut
1 tablespoon flaxseeds
1 teaspoon sesame seeds
1 tablespoon cocoa powder
1 teaspoon cinnamon
3 tablespoons almond butter
1 tablespoon tahini
2 teaspoons coconut palm sugar

Place all ingredients in a food processor and combine until the mixture begins to stick together. Roll the mixture into small balls, approximately 1 tablespoon each. Serve the treats right away or refrigerate them.

Coconut Banana Bread

(FOOD MATTERS)

YIELDS 6 SLICES

2 bananas, or at least 1 heaping cup of chopped bananas
4 fresh dates, pitted and chopped
4 medium organic free-range eggs
¼ cup coconut oil, melted
1 tablespoon pure maple syrup or raw honey
¾ cup coconut flour
½ teaspoon aluminum-free baking powder
¼ teaspoon unrefined sea salt
½ teaspoon ground cinnamon

Preheat the oven to 350°F.

In a bowl, mash the bananas with the chopped dates. (If the dates are quite dry and hard, soak them first in warm water.) In another bowl, whisk the eggs until they are fluffy, then combine them with the banana-date mash. Stir in the oil and maple syrup or honey. Add the flour, baking powder, salt, and cinnamon and combine well.

Transfer the batter to a loaf pan, greased and lined with parchment paper. The mixture will be quite thick, so flatten and smooth it with a rubber spatula. Bake for 35 to 40 minutes, or until a knife comes out clean when inserted and the bread's edges are browned.

Serve while warm, but allow the loaf to cool completely on a wire rack before storing any leftovers in an airtight container in the fridge.

Pumpkin Chocolate Chip Cookies

(FOOD MATTERS)

YIELDS 10 TO 15

1½ cups uncooked pumpkin flesh, cut into 1-inch cubes
¾ cup softened butter or melted coconut oil
½ cup pure maple syrup
1 teaspoon natural vanilla bean powder or extract
1¼ cups coconut flour or buckwheat flour
Pinch of baking powder (about ⅛ teaspoon)
1 teaspoon unrefined sea salt
2 teaspoons ground cinnamon
**¼ cup 70 to 85 percent dark chocolate chips, or chop a block
roughly into chunks**

Preheat the oven to 355°F.

Rub a couple of tablespoons of the softened butter or melted coconut oil over the pieces of pumpkin. Spread the pumpkin pieces on a baking sheet and roast them in the oven for 45 minutes, or until soft. Allow to cool slightly.

In a bowl, mix the cooked pumpkin, the remaining amount of butter or coconut oil, the maple syrup, and the vanilla. Sift in the flour, baking powder, salt, and cinnamon. Combine well to form a smooth batter. Then stir in the chocolate chips or chunks.

Onto a greased or parchment-lined baking sheet, spoon tablespoon-size rounds of the batter. Flatten these with the back of a spoon so that they are no more than ½-inch thick. Bake for about 15 to 20 minutes. They will still be soft, and the underside should be golden brown. Allow to cool completely on a wire rack before storing in an airtight container in the fridge.

Avocado Chocolate Mousse

(FOOD MATTERS)

SERVES 2

> **2 medium ripe avocados**
> **5 fresh dates, pitted and roughly chopped**
> **¼ cup coconut milk, nut milk, or filtered water**
> **⅓ cup raw cacao powder, or more to taste**
> **1 teaspoon natural vanilla extract or pure vanilla bean powder**
> **Pinch of unrefined sea salt**

Soak the dates in the milk or water for 10 to 30 minutes.

In a blender, place the avocado flesh, dates (along with their soaking milk or water), cacao powder, vanilla, and salt. Blend until smooth. You may need to add a little more liquid to facilitate blending. Scrape the sides of the blender down a few times during the process. Adjust ingredients to taste, adding more cacao powder if needed.

Transfer into two serving dishes and garnish with your choice of toppings, such as dried coconut, grated dark chocolate, or berries.

▶ By increasing the levels of specific neurotransmitters in our brains, cacao promotes a positive outlook, facilitates rejuvenation, and simply helps us feel good. Cacao beans are rich in a number of essential minerals, including magnesium, sulfur, calcium, iron, zinc, copper, potassium, and manganese.

Easy Fruit Ice Cream

(Jon Gabriel)

MAKES 4 KID-SIZE SERVINGS

> ¾ cup frozen fruit of your choice
> Pinch of stevia for raspberries or mixed berries (other fruits are
> naturally sweet enough)
> ⅔ cup plain yogurt
> 1 tablespoon ground flaxseeds

If the fruit is hard, allow it to soften for a few minutes. The fruit should be in small pieces rather than in one frozen block. Blend the fruit and the yogurt in a blender. Distribute the ice cream among four bowls, sprinkle with flaxseeds, and serve.

SNACKS AND DESSERTS

Easy Vanilla Ice Cream

(Jon Gabriel)

MAKES 2 KID-SIZE SERVINGS

> **2 frozen bananas, chopped**
> **¼ cup milk, Homemade Coconut Milk (page 125) or**
>   **Homemade Nut Milk (page 126) preferred**
> **1 teaspoon vanilla extract**
> **1 tablespoon ground flaxseeds**

Blend all the ingredients in a blender, then serve.

Easy Chocolate Ice Cream

(Jon Gabriel)

MAKES 2 KID-SIZE SERVINGS

> **2 frozen bananas, chopped**
> **¼ cup milk, Homemade Coconut Milk (page 125) or**
>   **Homemade Nut Milk (page 126) preferred**
> **4 teaspoons cocoa powder, raw preferred**
> **1 tablespoon ground flaxseeds**

Blend all the ingredients in a blender, then serve.

Simple Banana Ice Cream

(FOOD MATTERS)

SERVES 2

> **4 ripe bananas, peeled and roughly chopped**
> **½ cup filtered or spring water**

Freeze the bananas in a container for at least 12 hours. Put the frozen bananas in a blender with ¼ cup of the water, and blend until smooth and creamy. You may need to add up to ¼ cup more water to facilitate smooth blending.

Serve immediately in bowls or fill popsicle molds to have a treat on a stick!

Variations: You could add all sorts of things to this recipe. You could blend in ground cinnamon. Or add raw cacao powder and raw honey for a choc-banana ice cream. Vanilla extract tastes yummy too. Blending the bananas with kefir or yogurt adds beneficial bacteria.

▶ Always keep bananas in the freezer for a quick fix. Freeze any bananas that are on-the-turn, before they are overripe, rather than putting them to waste. Blending frozen bananas rather than fresh bananas, for either this recipe or in our smoothies, yields a much creamier, thicker texture.

Almond and Orange Cake

(Jon Gabriel)

SERVES 8

> **2 oranges**
> **1 ½ cups almonds**
> **6 medium organic free-range eggs**
> **½ cup coconut palm sugar**
> **1 teaspoon vanilla extract**

Grease an 8 × 8-inch cake pan and line the base with parchment paper.

Place the oranges, skins and all, in a large sauce pot. Cover them with water and bring to a boil. Once boiling, reduce the heat and simmer for approximately 30 minutes or until the skin has softened. Remove the oranges from the water and allow them to cool.

Preheat the oven to 300°F.

Chop the almonds in a food processor until they are coarsely chopped. Remove them from the food processor and set them aside.

Quarter the unpeeled oranges and place them in the food processor. Blend them at a low speed until smooth. Add the eggs one at a time. Then add the almonds, coconut palm sugar, and vanilla extract and continue to mix until combined.

Pour the mixture into the prepared pan and bake in the oven for approximately 1 hour and 15 minutes or until cooked through.

Chocolate Chia Crunch Brownies

(Jon Gabriel)

SERVES 8

1 cup ricotta cheese
5 tablespoons unsweetened cocoa powder, preferably raw
6 medium organic free-range egg yolks
4 tablespoons coconut sugar
½ tablespoon chia seeds
¼ cup walnuts or hazelnuts, crushed

Preheat the oven to 350°F. Grease a loaf pan and line it with parchment paper. Place all of the ingredients into a medium mixing bowl, and stir until well combined. Pour the mixture into the loaf pan and bake in the oven for 20 to 30 minutes. Check the brownies after 20 minutes by inserting a knife in the center of the brownies. Take the brownies out of the oven when the sides are cooked but the center is still slightly runny. Allow the brownies to sit for 15 minutes, then refrigerate them for 2 hours before serving.

Activated Nuts

(FOOD MATTERS)

Preparing nuts and seeds this way helps to make their minerals more bio-available (digestive), and it also makes them crispy and delicious to eat. Divide the quantities accordingly if you want to make smaller batches.

> **2 cups raw nuts or seeds (almonds, macadamia nuts, pecans, hazelnuts, Brazil nuts, pine nuts, pumpkin seeds, or sunflower seeds)**
> **Filtered or spring water, body-temperature warm, not cold**
> **1 teaspoon unrefined sea salt**

In a large bowl, place all of the ingredients with enough water to cover fully. Leave at room temperature for at least 4 hours, or overnight. Strain in a sieve. Store the nuts in a covered container in the fridge.

To keep for long periods, spread the nuts out in one layer over several baking sheets and dry them in an oven set at the lowest possible level, normally 112°F. Leave them until they are completely dried out and crunchy. This will take anywhere from 12 to 24 hours. Turn them several times during the drying process. Then store them in an airtight container.

▶ Why soak nuts? In traditional cultures, grains, seeds, and nuts were mostly soaked overnight, or for many days, to prepare them for consumption. Soaking grains and nuts activates the life-force energy within the seed and prepares it to germinate. Soaked and sprouted nuts contain more vitamins and minerals than unsoaked nuts.

Raw Vegetables with Satay Dip

(FOOD MATTERS)

SERVES 2 OR 3

> **3 celery stalks**
> **3 large carrots**
> **3 cucumbers**
> **1 red bell pepper**
> **1 tablespoon coconut oil**
> **1 teaspoon chili powder**
> **1 teaspoon curry powder**
> **1 cup coconut cream or milk (homemade if you have some)**
> **½ cup almond or peanut butter**

Cut the celery, carrots, cucumbers, and bell pepper into snack-size sticks and arrange on a serving platter.

In a small sauce pot, heat the coconut oil, chili powder, and curry powder and stir until fragrant (about 2 minutes). Stir in the coconut milk and almond or peanut butter. Once hot, and a creamy consistency is formed, the sauce is ready.

Serve the sauce in a small bowl placed in the middle of the platter of vegetables.

Three-Day Guided Detox

The goal of the Hungry for Change detox is to kick-start your health and assist you in making a transition to an overall healthier way of eating and living. This program is not the be-all and end-all of detox programs. Instead, think of it as a simple spring cleaning for your body. This detox will help reduce your cravings, reset your taste buds, start the process of cleaning up, and get you on the path to healthy living. The Hungry for Change detox offers an abundance of nutrient-rich whole foods and green juices, including delicious salads, soups, snacks, and desserts. So you definitely won't go hungry. The carefully selected ingredients will flood your body with nutrients, help flush out toxins, and keep you well hydrated.

We turn to this detox regularly and recommend it to our friends and family for three reasons: It's quick. It's easy to follow. And it doesn't require any hard-to-find ingredients or supplements. After the detox, you'll likely come away with increased energy, improved mental clarity, glowing skin, weight loss, increased immunity, and a renewed passion for life.

We recommend doing this detox twice a year, about once every six months. If you're feeling more adventurous or want to experience even better results, extend the detox to seven or ten days and add in some of the healthy lifestyle suggestions listed below. If you haven't done a detox before and are unsure what to expect, you might want to start the program on a Friday and complete the detox over the weekend. Some people may feel energized, others may want to rest; but either way, it's about listening to your body. Some people may experience mild detox symptoms, which include headaches, tiredness, irritability, and mucus elimination. These are all normal symptoms and a sign that your body is beginning to cleanse.

To download a printable version of this guide, which you can stick on your fridge, visit www.HungryForChange.tv/bonuses.

SIMPLE GROCERY LIST

1 large ginger root

1 head garlic

2 heads celery

1 large head kale

2 tubs mixed sprouts (alfalfa, sunflower, or watercress)

3 bunches parsley (curly leaf or flat leaf)

2 handfuls string beans

3 carrots

4 small zucchini

3 tomatoes

3 avocados

10 small cucumbers

3 pears (or apples)

6 lemons

3 handfuls raw almonds

4 ounces desiccated coconut for Homemade Coconut Milk (page 125) or, if you don't have a blender, 1 can of coconut milk or 1 carton almond or hemp milk

1 small jar ground cinnamon

1 packet chia seeds (enough for at least 4 tablespoons)

1 small packet toasted sesame seeds (enough for at least 3 tablespoons)

1 small package nori sheets (seaweed)

1 bottle naturally fermented wheat-free tamari or shoyu

Unrefined sea salt (or small tub of organic miso)

1 pack chamomile tea (whole leaves or tea bags—enough for at least 3 teas)

Barley grass or wheatgrass powder (optional)

Spirulina powder (optional)

Note: If a listed ingredient is not in season or available where you live, substitute something similar.

Ginger Lemon Detox Drink

Ginger is a powerful detoxifier that helps to kick-start your metabolism. Along with hydrating your body, this drink will help to stimulate bowel movements. Drink one large glass, but if you feel like more, go for it— hydration is important.

SERVES 1

> **1 12-ounce spring or filtered water, at room temperature**
> **Juice of ½ lemon**
> **½-inch knob of ginger root**

Add the lemon juice to the glass of water. Finely grate the ginger on a chopping board, then squeeze the ginger pieces in your hand, letting the juice of the ginger drip through your fingers and into the glass of water. Enjoy at room temperature upon rising for an amazing start to the day!

Super Detox Green Juice

This morning juice includes a potent blend of easily digestible alkaline minerals, such as potassium. Alkalizing your blood is important during the cleansing process because it keeps bad bacteria, yeast, and fungi in check, which helps keep cravings at bay. Drink one large glass, but feel free to have a second. If you don't have a juicer, try blending it up with some water. As an alternative, you could also try the Super Simple Green Drink (page 111).

SERVES 1

> **2 to 3 celery stalks, leaves removed**
> **1 small cucumber**
> **2 kale leaves**
> **Handful of fresh parsley**
> **1 small lemon or lime, peeled**
> **1 pear or apple**

Wash all of the ingredients and chop them so they can go through the juicer. Juice all of the ingredients and sip slowly.

For an extra health kick, stir in barley grass, wheatgrass, and/or spirulina powder.

Cucumber, Celery, and Carrot Sticks

This is your morning snack and keeps you on track with your cleanse. It's easy to prepare and carry with you when you're on the run.

SERVES 1

> **1 celery stalk, leaves removed**
> **1 small cucumber**
> **1 small carrot**

Wash all of the vegetables and cut them into small strips. Store in the fridge to keep them fresh and crisp.

Optionally, have another Super Detox Green Juice (page 245) or Super Simple Green Drink (page 111).

Sushi Salad

This salad includes a powerful mix of sprouts and sea vegetables. Sea vegetables, including nori, are one of the most nutrient-dense plant foods on the planet. They are particularly high in calcium and iodine, which helps to draw toxins from the body.

If you're at work or on the run, and have no time to prepare this salad, choose a big green vegetarian salad for lunch with an "all natural" dressing. Make sure to read the ingredients; if it looks suspect, ask for fresh lemon and extra-virgin olive oil on the side.

SERVES 1 OR 2

For the Dressing

1 tablespoon finely grated ginger root
1 tablespoon tamari or soy sauce
Juice of 1 lemon

For the Salad

1 ripe avocado, chopped
2 small cucumbers, halved and chopped
1 carrot, grated
Handful of sprouts (preferably alfalfa, watercress, or sunflower sprouts)
Handful of fresh cilantro, finely chopped
1 nori sheet, cut roughly with scissors into bite-size strips
1 tablespoon toasted sesame seeds

To prepare the dressing, take the ginger gratings and squeeze them between your fingers, making your hand a fist, into a small jar. Discard the pulp. Add the tamari (or soy sauce) and the lemon juice to the ginger juice. Close the lid and shake.

To prepare the salad, mix the avocado, cucumbers, carrot, sprouts, cilantro, and strips of nori together in a bowl and toss with the salad dressing. Sprinkle seeds over the top to garnish.

Activated Almonds

Soaked or activated nuts will be your afternoon snack throughout this cleanse. Plan ahead by soaking a large bowl of raw almonds overnight, straining the water away in the morning, and storing them covered in the fridge.

2 cups raw nuts or seeds (almonds, macadamia nuts, pecans, hazelnuts, Brazil nuts, pine nuts, pumpkin seeds, or sunflower seeds)
Filtered or spring water, at room temperature
1 teaspoon unrefined sea salt

In a large bowl, place all of the ingredients with enough water to cover fully. Leave at room temperature for at least 4 hours, or overnight. Strain in a sieve. Store the nuts in a covered container in the fridge.

Potassium Balance Soup

Based on a recipe from physician Henry Bieler (Bieler's Broth), this vegetable tonic provides an ideal combination for restoring acid–alkaline and sodium–potassium balance to the body's organs and glands.

SERVES 3 (1 SERVING PER NIGHT DURING THE DETOX)

>   **4 cups spring or filtered water**
>   **4 medium zucchini, finely chopped**
>   **3 celery stalks, leaves removed, then finely chopped**
>   **1 cup roughly chopped green string beans**
>   **1 large bunch fresh parsley, stems and leaves roughly chopped**
>   **3 medium tomatoes, finely chopped**
>   **3 garlic cloves, finely chopped**
>   **2 teaspoons unrefined sea salt or 1 tablespoon organic miso paste**
>   **2 teaspoons dried thyme, rosemary, oregano, or other French**
>   **Provence herbs for added flavor**

Put all of the ingredients in a large stock or sauté pot. Bring to a gentle boil, then lower the heat, cover, and let simmer gently for 30 minutes. Serve warm.

If you wish to create a thicker soup, you can purée the soup in batches in a blender or blend it with an immersion, or "stick," blender until smooth and creamy; however, this soup is also delicious as is.

Store covered in the fridge for use within one week, or freeze for extended storage.

Chia Seed Pudding Recipe

This after-dinner snack includes chia seeds, a gelatinous plant food that helps to draw out toxins from the liver and pass them into the colon for excretion. Chia seeds are also high in omega-3 and make you feel full and satiated!

SERVES 3 (1 SERVING PER NIGHT DURING THE DETOX)

> 1¼ cups Homemade Nut Milk (page 126) or Homemade Coconut Milk (page 125), or if you don't have time, use store-bought almond or hemp milk
>
> 1 tablespoon raw honey or maple syrup
>
> 4 tablespoons chia seeds
>
> 1 teaspoon ground cinnamon

In a large jar, combine all of the ingredients and shake well. Pour the mixture into 3 small bowls or glasses and refrigerate until it thickens into a pudding-like consistency, about 30 minutes. This is a delicious treat and keeps for up to a week, covered in the fridge.

Calming Chamomile Tea

Chamomile tea will help to calm your body and prepare you for a restful night's sleep. Deep restful sleep during this cleanse is important because of how it will help you digest unwanted stress hormones, which can cause you to gain weight.

SERVES 1

> **1 cup spring or filtered water**
> **1 chamomile tea bag or 1 tablespoon dried chamomile flowers**

Bring the water to a boil and pour into a teacup or mug. Add the tea bag or, if using loose flowers, use a teapot and a strainer. Steep for 3 to 5 minutes, then enjoy.

Optionally, try other herbal detox teas, such as nettle, dandelion root, or licorice root.

Evening Affirmation and Visualization

Your positive affirmation during this detox is "I accept myself unconditionally right now!" Say this out loud to yourself in the mirror before going to bed or whenever you find time throughout your day.

Also, just before you go to sleep, practice your evening visualization by envisioning the body and health you most desire. Download a guided visualization MP3 with Jon Gabriel at www.HungryForChange.tv/bonuses.

Healthy Lifestyle Tips

During the Hungry for Change detox, try to clear your calendar and look after yourself as much as possible. Keep the distractions to a minimum. This includes TV, Facebook, business appointments, or anything else that might divide your attention. To get the most out of the cleanse, it's important that you are in a supportive environment and remain in a relaxed state.

The suggestions below will aid the body's natural detoxification processes and boost your mood and energy levels. You'll feel so good, you'll want to incorporate them into your new healthy lifestyle!

Exercise: Exercise and movement are a very important part of the cleansing process. They improve circulation and help expel toxins and relax the body. Go for a brisk thirty-minute walk at a place you feel is the most pleasant, such as the beach or a nice park.

Be in nature: Fresh air and sunshine support the cleansing and oxygenation of cells and tissues and help revitalize our bodies. Be careful to avoid excessive exposure to the sun.

Sauna: *Enjoy an infrared sauna or steam room, to increase circulation and to assist the elimination of toxins through the skin.*

Yoga: *Before your main meal, try thirty minutes or an hour of yoga. Start with some sun salutations and include a shoulder stand, which stimulates the thyroid gland and regulates metabolism. (If you're not familiar with these poses, Google them. They're easy to learn and fun to practice.)*

Breathing: *Take ten deep breaths three times a day. Inhale for a count of four, hold for a count of eight, and exhale for a count of sixteen. Use your diaphragm so that your stomach expands as you inhale. As you exhale, visualize it as a detoxifying breath.*

Skin brushing: *Before you hop in the shower, brush your skin from head to toe, using small, quick strokes. Use a soft-bristled skin brush, which is available for purchase at most health food stores or pharmacies. Brushing your skin for five minutes a day helps increase circulation and break down fatty deposits within your body.*

Massage: *Get a massage. Any type of body massage will help get your blood flowing. If time or money is a concern, try a reflexology foot massage, which helps stimulate the body's detoxification organs.*

Bathing: *Take a steamy bath and exfoliate your body with a loofah. Add Epsom salts or bentonite clay to the water for extra detoxification benefits.*

Meditation: *Begin the day with a fifteen-minute meditation. Sit quietly and focus on your breathing. Visualize your body detoxifying. As you inhale, visualize healthy oxygen entering your lungs and bloodstream. As you exhale, visualize toxins leaving the body.*

Avoiding stimulants: *Avoid stimulants like coffee, black teas, alcohol, cigarettes, and sweets. Sip on herbal teas or lemon water to help fire up the liver's waste-elimination process.*

Hydration: *Drink lots of fresh spring or filtered water (up to two liters per day) to help flush the system. It is important not to drink water with meals as water dilutes the digestive enzymes, preventing the body from assimilating nutrients. Drink water thirty minutes before eating, then allow one hour or more after eating before drinking again.*

Go natural: *Use natural body-care products, including natural toothpastes, body lotions, and deodorants. These products should be free of sodium lauryl sulfate, sodium laureth sulfate, aluminum, and fluoride. A good rule of thumb: If you can't eat it, then you shouldn't put it on your body.*

Colon cleanse: *For those wishing to try something new, schedule a colonic, or colon irrigation. A colonic session removes the mucoidal plaque that may line the walls of your colon. After a colonic, some people notice their stomach area appears slightly more flat. If a colonic does not appeal to you but you still want to cleanse the colon, then you can give yourself an enema at home. Most pharmacies or drugstores will sell enema kits, which will help to clear out your bowels. Make sure you take a high-quality probiotic supplement after any enema or colonic. This will help to replace any good bacteria lost from your colon cleanse. Your colonic hydrotherapist, health food store nutritionist, or naturopath will be able to advise you.*

Profile in Health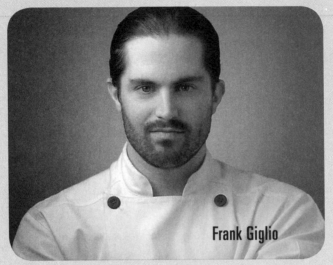

Frank Giglio

Having spent more than fifteen years in the culinary field, I feel like I have come a long way in my own personal journey and adapted cuisine. As a young culinary student, I was far from informed on the importance of creating and eating well-balanced, nutritious meals. Nobody told me about the dangers of refined and overly processed foods.

Lucky for me, I watched my health decline, my weight incline, and my spirits hit an all-time low. Lucky because I needed to feel terrible in order to truly want to feel great! Eventually I completely overhauled my diet and lifestyle and immediately felt the difference. This profound change enabled me to continue to educate myself so that I could continue to teach and inspire others to live the best life they can.

I eat a lot of different foods. As my friend Daniel Vitalis mentions in his lectures, I eat from the Four Kingdoms. I eat plants, animals, fungi, and bacteria. Depending on the time of the year, or specific health goal I may have, I sometimes eat a lot from one kingdom and less from another. Overall, though, my diet is all about finding the proper balance among the Four Kingdoms. Nature drives me, and I choose to eat as much food from the forest as I can. I love wild foods and I love herbs, so I find it essential to add them to my cuisine.

On pages 258–59, you will find comprehensive seven-day meal plans that I think will help increase your health. More than anything, I feel that the willingness to learn—and keeping an open mind—will lead you in the right direction.

Best in health,
Frank Giglio

❭ Frank Giglio fell in love with the fascinating world of food at the age of fifteen. Eager and intrigued, he began apprenticing directly under some of the top chefs in the United States, who instilled in him a deep understanding of the creative process in working with food and infused in him the importance of fine arts mastery, since tastes and flavors inspire an artistic passion for creating delicious and nourishing cuisine. A graduate of the Institute for Integrative Nutrition in New York City, he trained as a chef at the New England Culinary Institute in Montpelier, Vermont. While his culinary offerings are based in classic technique and traditional food preparation, he also uses food as medicine. Wearing his chef's hat, he focuses on sustainable cuisine, seeking the highest quality foods, grown locally and harvested in season, and supporting the crucial farm-to-table method of preparing food. He remains deeply connected to the earth in his daily life, merging herbalism and living-food nutrition with wild-food foraging. He creates innovative dishes that are wholesome and full of vitality and have a very small ecological footprint. He feels blessed to be able to share this passion with his clients, and with his wife and their young son.

Seven-Day Meal Plan

Frank Giglio

Monday
Breakfast: Creamy Blueberry Smoothie (page 127)
Lunch: Quinoa Salad with Fragrant Spices (page 187)
Dinner: Scrumptious Burger Salad with Lemon-Herb Vinaigrette (page 185)

Tuesday
Breakfast: Build-Your-Own Breakfast Cereal (page 148)
Lunch: Wild Salmon Collard Wraps (page 206)
Dinner: French Onion Soup (page 159)

Wednesday
Breakfast: Veggie Frittata (page 145)
Lunch: Red Lentil and Coconut Curry Dhal (page 163)
Dinner: Roasted Tempeh with Shiitake and Sweet Potato (page 199)

Thursday
Breakfast: Homegrown Granola (page 150)
Lunch: Asian-Inspired Quinoa Salad (page 181)
Dinner: Curry-Spiced Fish Cakes with Mango Salsa (page 208)

Friday
Breakfast: Poached Eggs over Sautéed Greens (page 147)
Lunch: Steamed Cauliflower and Broccoli with Chunky Avocado Salad (page 170)
Dinner: Chinese Salmon Salad (page 183)

Saturday
Breakfast: Warm Breakfast Porridge (page 152)
Lunch: Big Ole Garden Salad (page 174)
Dinner: Slow-Cooked Chicken Thighs (page 220)

Sunday
Breakfast: Kickin' Breakfast Burritos (page 155)
Lunch: Mineral-Rich Raw Green Soup (page 158)
Dinner: Shrimp and Kale Sauté (page 212)

Vegetarian Seven-Day Meal Plan

James Colquhoun, Laurentine ten Bosch, and Frank Giglio

Monday
Breakfast: Refreshing Cucumber, Pear, and Fennel Juice and Perfect Scrambled Eggs (pages 110 and 144)
Lunch: Skin Beauty Salad (page 173)
Dinner: Omelet Pizza (page 200)

Tuesday
Breakfast: Super Simple Green Drink and Millet Porridge (pages 111 and 151)
Lunch: Blueberry Salad with Lemon Ginger Dressing (page 172)
Dinner: French Onion Soup (page 159)

Wednesday
Breakfast: Ginger Lemon Detox Drink and Veggie Frittata (pages 113 and 145)
Lunch: Red Lentil and Coconut Curry Dhal (page 163)
Dinner: Zucchini Alfredo Without Dairy (page 191)

Thursday
Breakfast: Berry Kefir Smoothie and Homegrown Granola (pages 137 and 150)
Lunch: Asian-Inspired Quinoa Salad (page 181)
Dinner: Egg and Lemon Soup with Quinoa (page 162)

Friday
Breakfast: Ginger Lemon Tea and Poached Eggs over Sautéed Greens (pages 141 and 147)
Lunch: Steamed Cauliflower and Broccoli with Chunky Avocado Salad (page 170)
Dinner: Roasted Vegetable Salad with Yogurt Dressing (page 180)

Saturday
Breakfast: Super Simple Green Drink and Warm Breakfast Porridge (pages 111 and 152)
Lunch: Big Ole Garden Salad (page 174)
Dinner: Veggie Fritters and Greens with Almond and Lemon (pages 192 and 201)

Sunday
Breakfast: Kickin' Breakfast Burritos (page 155)
Lunch: Mineral-Rich Raw Green Soup (page 158)
Dinner: Strawberry, Pecan, and Goat Cheese Salad and Sweet Potato Fries (pages 171 and 193)

The Dirty Dozen
and Clean Fifteen

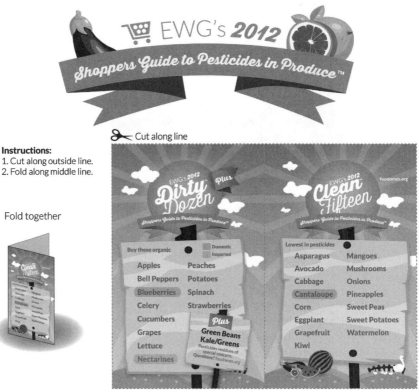

Instructions:
1. Cut along outside line.
2. Fold along middle line.

Fold together

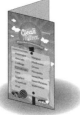

✂ Cut along line

EWG's 2012
Shoppers Guide to Pesticides in Produce™

EWG's 2012 — Dirty Dozen *Plus*
Shoppers Guide to Pesticides in Produce™

Buy these organic — Domestic / Imported

Apples	Peaches
Bell Peppers	Potatoes
Blueberries	Spinach
Celery	Strawberries
Cucumbers	
Grapes	**Plus**
Lettuce	**Green Beans**
Nectarines	**Kale/Greens**

Pesticides residues of special concern. Questions? foodnews.org

EWG's 2012 — Clean Fifteen
Shoppers Guide to Pesticides in Produce™

foodnews.org

Lowest in pesticides

Asparagus	Mangoes
Avocado	Mushrooms
Cabbage	Onions
Cantaloupe	Pineapples
Corn	Sweet Peas
Eggplant	Sweet Potatoes
Grapefruit	Watermelon
Kiwi	

Recommended Reading

Clean: The Revolutionary Program to Restore the Body's Natural Ability to Heal Itself (expanded edition) by Dr. Alejandro Junger. San Francisco: HarperOne, 2012.

The Wisdom of Menopause: Creating Physical and Emotional Health During the Change (revised edition) by Dr. Christiane Northrup. New York: Bantam Books, 2012.

Women's Bodies, Women's Wisdom: Creating Physical and Emotional Health and Healing (revised edition) by Dr. Christiane Northrup. New York: Bantam Books, 2010.

Eating for Beauty by David Wolfe. Berkeley, CA: North Atlantic Books, 2003.

Take Control of Your Health by Dr. Joseph Mercola and Dr. Kendra Pearsall. Mercola.com, 2007.

Sweet Deception: Why Splenda, NutraSweet, and the FDA May Be Hazardous to Your Health by Dr. Joseph Mercola and Dr. Kendra Pearsall. Nashville: Thomas Nelson Books, 2006.

Slim for Life: Freedom from the Diet Trap by Jason Vale. London: Thorsons Publishers, 2008.

Juice Yourself Slim: Lose Weight Without Dieting by Jason Vale. London: Thorsons Publishers, 2008.

The Gabriel Method: The Revolutionary Diet-Free Way to Lose Weight by Jon Gabriel. Cammeray, Australia: Simon & Schuster, 2009.

Crazy Sexy Diet: Eat Your Veggies, Ignite Your Spark, and Live Like You Mean It! by Kris Carr. Guilford, CT: Skirt!, 2011.

Crazy Sexy Cancer Tips by Kris Carr. Guilford, CT: Skirt!, 2007.

Fat, Sick & Nearly Dead by Joe Cross. Blurb, 2011.

The Hormone Factor by Ralph Moorman (digital book). 2010.

No Grain Diet: Conquer Carbohydrate Addiction and Stay Slim for Life by Dr. Joseph Mercola. New York: Plume, 2004.

Your Body's Many Cries for Water by Dr. F. Batmanghelidj. Falls Church, VA: Global Health Solutions, 2008.

Superfoods: The Food and Medicine of the Future by David Wolfe. Berkeley, CA: North Atlantic Books, 2009.

Doctor Yourself: Natural Healing That Works by Andrew Saul. Basic Health Publications, 2003.

The Gerson Therapy: The Proven Nutritional Program for Cancer and Other Illnesses by Charlotte Gerson and Morton Walker, D.P.M. New York: Kensington, 2001.

Apple Cider Vinegar: Miracle Health Systems by Patricia Bragg and Paul C. Bragg. Santa Barbara, CA: Bragg Health Sciences, 2008.

Deep Nutrition: Why Your Genes Need Traditional Food by Dr. Catherine Shanahan and Luke Shanahan. Big Box Books, 2008.

The Cholesterol Myths: Exposing the Fallacy That Saturated Fat and Cholesterol Cause Heart Disease by Uffe Ravnskov. Warsaw, IN: New Trends Publishing, 2002.

Food Is Better Medicine Than Drugs: Your Prescription for Drug-Free Health by Patrick Holford and Jerome Burne. London: Piatkus Books, 2007.

Healthy Healing: A Guide to Self-Healing for Everyone by Dr. Linda Page. Healthy Healing Inc., 2004.

Body Ecology Diet: Recovering Your Health and Rebuilding Your Immunity by Donna Gates. New York and London: Hay House, 2011.

Nutrition and Physical Degeneration by Weston Price, D.D.S. Lemon-Grove, CA: Price-Pottenger Nutrition Foundation, 2008.

The Blood Sugar Solution: The UltraHealthy Program for Losing Weight, Preventing Disease, and Feeling Great Now! by Dr. Mark Hyman. New York: Little, Brown, 2012.

Jamie at Home: Cook Your Way to the Good Life by Jamie Oliver. New York: Hyperion, 2008.

Food Rules: An Eater's Manual by Michael Pollan. New York: Penguin, 2010.

Heal Your Body A–Z: The Mental Causes for Physical Illness and the Way to Overcome Them by Louise Hay. New York and London: Hay House, 1998.

The Teachers

The *HUNGRY FOR CHANGE* book would not have been possible without the incredible contributions from the following teachers. These people have dedicated their lives and professions to helping people improve their health, and for that we are eternally grateful.

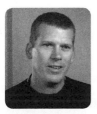

Mike Adams is a natural-health author and award-winning journalist with a strong interest in personal health, the environment, and the power of nature to help us heal. He has authored more than 1,800 articles and dozens of reports, guides, and interviews on natural-health topics, impacting the lives of millions of readers around the world. Also known as the Health Ranger, Mike Adams is the founder and editor of NaturalNews.com.

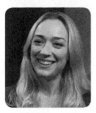

Kris Carr is the *New York Times* bestselling author of *Crazy Sexy Diet, Crazy Sexy Cancer Tips, Crazy Sexy Cancer Survivor,* and *Crazy Sexy Kitchen*. A motivational speaker and wellness coach, she leads workshops at wellness centers throughout the United States and lectures at medical schools, hospitals, and universities. Kris has been featured on *The Today Show, Good Morning America, The CBS Evening News, The Gayle King Show,* and *The Oprah Winfrey Show*. She is the founder of the award-winning online magazine *Crazy Sexy Life* at crazysexylife.com.

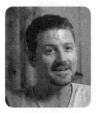

Joe Cross is the director of *Fat, Sick, and Nearly Dead,* a documentary about regaining his health, and founder of Reboot Your Life, a lifestyle brand that provides information, tools, consumer products, and community support that encourage people to consume more fruits and vegetables in order to improve their health and vitality. His website is www.jointhereboot.com.

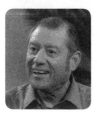

Harvey Diamond, a pioneer in helping shift people toward healthier eating, is a health and wellness advocate and *New York Times* bestselling author. His Fit for Life books have sold nearly 14 million copies and have been translated into 33 different languages. His website is harveydiamond.com.

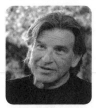

Frank Ferrante is the subject of the documentary *May I Be Frank*. A lover of life, great food, beautiful women, and a good laugh, Frank was also a drug addict, morbidly obese, prediabetic, and fighting hepatitis C. *May I Be Frank* documents the transformation of Frank Ferrante's life. His website is mayibefrankferrante.com.

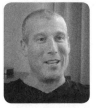

Jon Gabriel, a weight-loss and visualization expert, is the bestselling author of *The Gabriel Method*. In 1990 Jon started gaining weight for no apparent reason. He tried every diet and program he could to lose weight, but in the end, he just kept gaining. The more he dieted, the more he gained. The situation became critical in mid-2001 when he became morbidly obese and reached a weight of over 410 pounds. Jon lost over 220 pounds without dieting and without surgery. His website is www.GabrielMethod.com.

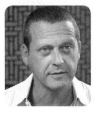

Alejandro Junger, M.D., is the *New York Times* bestselling author of *Clean*. Born in Uruguay, Dr. Junger graduated from medical school there in 1990 and moved to New York City for his postgraduate training. He completed his training in internal medicine at New York University Downtown Hospital and his fellowship in cardiology at Lenox Hill Hospital in New York City. His drastic change in lifestyle and diet from his move to New York City soon manifested as irritable bowel syndrome and depression. Becoming a patient of the system he was practicing was such a shock that it started a journey to search for an alternative solution to his health problems. His website is www.cleanprogram.com.

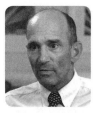

Dr. Joseph Mercola is an osteopathic physician whose passion lies in transforming the traditional medical paradigm in the United States. Named the Ultimate Wellness Game Changer by *The Huffington Post* in 2009, he is the author of *Sweet Deception* and the *New York Times* bestselling books *The Great Bird Flu Hoax* and *The No-Grain Diet*. He is the founder of Mercola.com.

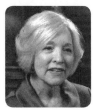

Christiane Northrup, M.D., is the world's leading authority on women's health and wellness. A board-certified ob-gyn physician who graduated from Dartmouth Medical School and did her residency at Tufts–New England Medical Center, Dr. Northrup was also an assistant clinical professor of obstetrics-gynecology at Maine Medical Center for twenty years. Recognizing the unity of body, mind, and spirit, she helps empower women to tune in to their innate inner wisdom to positively transform their health. She is the author of the *New York Times* bestselling books *Women's Bodies, Women's Wisdom* and *The Wisdom of Menopause*. Her website is www.drnorthrup.com.

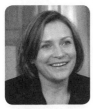

Evita Ramparte is a leading health journalist, holistic coach, and media producer. She transformed her health through juicing and a plant-based diet after an ovarian cancer diagnosis in 2000. She's been interviewed by MTV Europe and *Cosmopolitan* magazine, and she empowers people to transform their own health. Her website is www .evitaramparte.com.

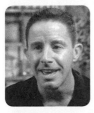

Jason Vale is a leading authority on health, addiction, and juicing. His books—7*lbs in 7 Days: Super Juice Diet, Juice Master: Turbo-Charge Your Life in 14 Days*, and *Slim for Life*—have sold more than 2 million copies around the world. Jason turned to juicing to transform his own health and is now known as the Juice Master. He helps transform people's health the world over through his books, DVDs, and juice retreats. His website is www.thejuicemaster.com.

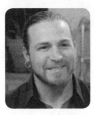

Daniel Vitalis is a nature-based philosopher and a leading health, nutrition, and personal development strategist. He is a leading traditional- and wild-foods expert and teaches that invincible health is a product of living in alignment with our biological design and our role in the ecosystem. His website is www.danielvitalis.com.

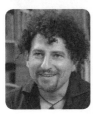

David Wolfe is one of the world's leading authorities on super foods and nutrition. He holds a master's in nutrition and is the author of *Eating for Beauty; The Sunfood Diet Success System; Naked Chocolate; David Wolfe on Raw Foods, Superfoods, and Superherbs; Superfoods: The Food and Medicine of the Future;* and *The Longevity NOW Program.* His website is www.davidwolfe.com.

Credits

Grateful acknowledgment is made for permission to include (and in some cases to reprint) information and recipes:

Information about unhealthy diets on pages 15 and 16 courtesy of Mike Adams.

Information about chemicals in cosmetics on pages 86 and 87 courtesy of the David Suzuki Foundation.

Information about superfoods on page 53 and eating for beauty on page 90 courtesy of David Wolfe.

Recipe on page 131 is reproduced by permission of Mike Adams.

Recipes on pages 112, 114, 120, 121, and 122 are reproduced by permission of Joe Cross.

Recipes on pages 109, 130, 132, 134, 135, 156, 161, 175, 176, 177, 178, 192, 200, 201, 215, 221, 229, 233, 234, 235, 237, and 238 are reproduced by permission of Jon Gabriel.

Recipes on pages 127, 145, 147, 148, 150, 152, 155, 158, 159, 163, 165, 166, 167, 168, 170, 174, 181, 183, 185, 187, 199, 202, 203, 204, 205, 206, 208, 212, and 220 are used with permission of Frank Giglio.

Recipes on pages 153, 154, 194, 195, 196, 197, 198, 211, 213, and 214 are reproduced by permission of Dr. Joseph Mercola, D.O.

Recipes on pages 115, 116, 117, 118, 119, 123, 124, 128, 129, 133, 136, 138, 184, and 186 are reproduced by permission of Jason Vale.

Recipe on page 142 is reproduced by permission of Daniel Vitalis.

Recipes on pages 108, 110, 111, 113, 125, 126, 137, 139, 140, 141, 143, 144, 146, 149, 151, 157, 160, 162, 164, 169, 171, 172, 173, 179, 180, 182, 188, 189, 190, 191, 193, 207, 209, 210, 216, 218, 222, 223, 224, 226, 228, 230, 231, 232, 236, 239, and 240 are reproduced by permission of James Colquhoun, Laurentine ten Bosch, and Emma Sgourakis, *FOOD MATTERS: The Recipe Book.*

Acknowledgments

Special thanks to:

Dr. Alejandro Junger
Dr. Christiane Northrup
David Wolfe
Daniel Vitalis
Dr. Joseph Mercola
Jason Vale
Jon Gabriel
Kris Carr
Mike Adams
Evita Ramparte
Frank Ferrante
Joe Cross
Jamie Oliver
Siddha Yoga Foundation
Connect with Spirit
Harvey Diamond
Ralph Moorman
Nick Ortner
Sue Dengate
Rory Freedman
Philip McCluskey
Dr. Romeo Brooks
Gideon Weil
Miles Doyle
Suzanne Quist
Babette Dunkelgrun
Melinda Mullin
Terri Leonard
Mark Tauber
Claudia Boutote
Laina Adler
Enzo Tedeschi
David Sander

Carlo Ledesma
Carla Nirella
Frank Giglio
Anthony Robbins
Jamie Oliver
Oprah Winfrey
Roy and Megan Colquhoun
Karian and Berend ten Bosch
Oma Hetty ten Bosch
Oma Ditty Zwollo
Janharm and Cinda Musters
Allen Adkins
Alex and Karen Ortner
Nick Ortner
Monika Lopez
Kipp Stroden
Christina Afentoulis
Chip Grey
Buck Palmer and Ashley Hart
Georgie Pierce
Jocelyn Musters
Emma Sgourakis
Nigel Hall
Michael Maidens
Corrina McGowan
Rachel Morrow
Harmony Parkes
Belinda Pooley
Patrick Walsh
Russell, Matt, Tom
    and the team at OMC
Jonathan Weyland
Jany and Michel Blanchard
Chase Carter
John Butler Trio

Index

teas and hot drinks *(continued)*
   Coconut Chai, 143
   Ginger Lemon Tea, 141
   Ginger Turmeric Detox Tea, 139
   Happy Hot Chocolate, 140
   Health Elixir Tea, 142
teenagers
   consumption of sugar, xi–xii
   fructose consumption, 24
   pre-diabetes and diabetes in, xiii
Tempeh, Roasted, with Shiitake and
   Sweet Potato, 199
ten nutritional tips, 44–48
ten Bosch, Laurentine, *1*, 3–6, 80
Thai Coconut Soup, 160
Three-Day Guided Detox, 241–52
   after dinner tea, 251
   afternoon snack, 248
   before bed affirmation and
     visualization, 252
   breakfast, 245
   dessert, 250
   dinner, 249
   drink upon rising, 244
   lunch, 247
   mid-morning snack, 246
   printable guide, 242
   simple grocery list, 243
thyroid gland, 52
   kale caution, 223
tomato(es), 90
   Big Ole Garden Salad, 174
   Bruschetta Juice, 120
   Chili, 221
   Chili Mussels, 215
   Gazpacho Juice, 122
   Kickin' Breakfast Burritos, 155
   Mineral-Rich Raw Green Soup, 158
   Potassium Balance Soup, 249
   Salad in a Glass, 123
   Veggie Frittata, 145
torula yeast, 32
toxins
   artificial sweeteners, 22–23
   chemical contamination, 95–97
   expelling, through the skin, 88
   expelling, water and, 60

   in food containers, 16
   plastics and petrochemicals, 18
   skin absorption of, 18, 85
   in skin creams and cosmetics, 85,
     86–87
   what to avoid completely, 104
trans fats, xii, xiii, 193
triclosan, 87
trout, 30
Tuna, Asian-Flavored, with Stir-Fried
   Vegetables, 204
turmeric
   Ginger, Detox Tea, 139
   Quinoa Salad with Fragrant Spices,
     187
turnip greens, 98

U.S. Department of Agriculture
   (USDA), 15

Vale, Jason, 19–20, 21, 25, 30, 37, 55–56,
   92, 92–93
vegetables. *See also* greens; *specific types*
   Asian-Flavored Tuna with Stir-Fried,
     204
   recommended percentage of diet, xi
   recommended servings daily, 44
   Roasted, Salad with Yogurt Dressing,
     180
   Veggie Delight, 115
   Veggie Frittata, 145
   Veggie Fritters, 192
vinegars
   Avocado with Raw Apple Cider
     Vinegar, 222
   raw apple cider, 51, 63
visualization, 71–73, *72*
   before bed, 252
   best times to practice, 73
   guided, with Jon Gabriel, 252
   morning, 254
Vitalis, Daniel, 12, *17*, 17–18, 37, 48,
   50–51, 60–61, 83, 97, 98–99, 104, 256
   website, 18
vitamins, 14
   A, 14, 144
   B12, 144

B complex, 14
C, 14, 56, 89
D, 14, 84, 144
E, 14, 144
K, 14, 144

walnuts
  Homegrown Granola, 150
water
  best type to drink, 61, 63
  chronic dehydration and, 60
  hydrating, 255
  lack of, in American diet, 15
  quality of, 60–61
  as source of life, 60–62
  toxins in, 61
watercress, 52, 90
Watermelon Crush, 134
weight gain, 6
  artificial sweeteners and, 32
  dieting and, 36, 39–40
  hunter-gatherer-gardener ancestors
    and, 11
  lack of vitamin D and, 84
  "liquid pounds," 70
  sleep deprivation and, 70
  stress and, 11–12, 67–69
  sugar and, 26
  trans fats and, xiii
weight loss. *See also* Profiles in Health
  adding in good stuff strategy, 38
  detoxification and, 96
  diet trap, 29–40
  emotional eating and, 67–80
  foods from healthy sources and, 104
  nutrient dense diet and, xiv, 7
  probiotics and, 51
  seaweeds for, 52
  self-love and, 73–80, 74, 76, 77,
    78, 79

stress and, 70
visualization and, 71–73, 72
vitamin D and, 84
why diets don't work, 36–37
wheatgrass, 52
  Super Simple Green Drink, 111
whole grains, xiv
  gluten-free types, 46
  gluten in, reducing, 45–46
  soaking, 151
Wild Salmon Collard Wraps, 206
wines, 51
Wolfe, David, 38, 51–52, 53, 64, 83, 85,
    88, 97
  tips on eating for beauty, 90
  Top 10 Superfoods, 53
  website, 53

yeast extract, 21, 32, 47
yoga, 254
yogurt, 51, 64
  Breakfast on the Move, 128
  Creamy Blueberry Smoothie, 127
  Protein Power Smoothie, 129
  Spirulina Breakfast Smoothie, 130
"You are what you eat," 5, 15, 43–44

zinc, 90, 232
zucchini
  Asian-Flavored Tuna with Stir-Fried
    Vegetables, 204
  Instant Green Soup for One, 164
  Mushroom Soup, 165
  Potassium Balance Soup, 249
  Raw, Dairy-Free Alfredo, 191
  Roasted Vegetable Salad with Yogurt
    Dressing, 180
  Sunshine in a Glass, 116
  Veggie Delight, 115
  Veggie Frittata, 145

Discover the Film

To watch *HUNGRY FOR CHANGE:*
A Documentary Film About Lasting Weight Loss,
Abundant Energy, and Vibrant Health,
visit your local DVD retailer, Amazon, iTunes,
NetFlix, or www.HungryForChange.tv.

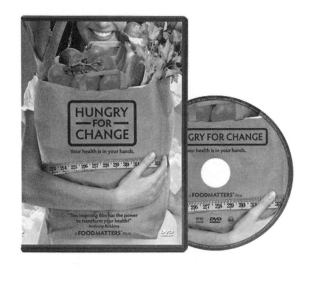

Download Your Free Bonuses

To download your free bonuses
to help keep you motivated and apply all
of the knowledge from the book, visit
www.HungryForChange.tv/bonuses.

Scan this code with your smartphone to be linked to *HUNGRY FOR CHANGE* bonus materials on the Elixir mobile site, where you'll also find information about other healthy living books and related materials!

You can also text keyword CHANGE to READIT (732348) to be sent a link to the mobile website.